A Social History of Medicine

Themes in British Social History

Edited by Dr J. Stevenson

The Englishman's Health
Poverty in the Sixteenth and Seventeenth Centuries
Popular Protest and Public Order 1750–1939
Religion and Society in Industrial England
Religion and Society in Tudor England
Sex, Politics and Social Change
A Social History of Medicine
Leisure and Society 1830–1950
The Army and Society 1815–1914

A Social History of Medicine

Frederick F. Cartwright

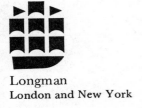

Longman
London and New York

Longman Group Limited London

*Associated companies, branches and representatives
throughout the world*

*Published in the United States of America
by Longman Inc., New York*

First published 1977

Library of Congress Cataloging in Publication Data

Cartwright, Frederick Fox.
    A social history of medicine.

    (Themes in British social history)
    Bibliography: p.
    1. Medicine—Great Britain—History.   2. Social
medicine—Great Britain—History.   I. Title.
[DNLM: 1. History of medicine—Great Britain.
WZ70 FA1 C3s]
R487.C37   362.1'0941   76-41898
ISBN 0 582 48393 X
ISBN 0 582 48394 8 pbk.

Set in IBM Baskerville 9 on 11pt
and printed in Great Britain by
Richard Clay (The Chaucer Press) Ltd,
Bungay

Contents

Acknowledgements

Cover illustrations:

We wish to thank the Radio Times, Hulton Picture Library, for permission to reproduce two illustrations the first of which depicts *Free Medical Attention for Children—Cleansing Station 1912*; the second shows the *East London Hospital for Children—1878 Princess Mary Ward*; and Professor R. R. Gillies for a photograph showing a *Primary Syphilitic Chancre*.

A Social History of Medicine

1 The philosophy of medicine before Rudolf Virchow and Louis Pasteur

The primary purpose of a social history of medicine must be to describe how the practice of medicine has affected the health and development of people. But practice, that is diagnosis and treatment, depends upon theory. From the earliest times the orthodox physician has sought a tenable theory of causes, the reason or reasons why disease occurs. This is the philosophy of medicine. Our first chapter will deal not so much with medicine as it affected people but with the development of a philosophy upon which the practice was based. This necessarily brief and incomplete survey of changing ideas will be followed into the nineteenth century when the work of such men as Rudolf Virchow, Louis Pasteur, Charles Darwin and Gregor Mendel changed medicine from an empiric art into a rational science.

Primitive man supposed both disease and cure to be effected by a supernatural agency, malign or beneficent. A bad spirit might cause pestilence, a good spirit achieve its cure. Thus the 'orthodox physician' could be priest or anti-priest. In both cases he would be a particularly gifted or skilled person, the priest capable of interceding with the god or of overcoming the devil, the anti-priest partaking of devildom and so possessing a special knowledge of how the evil spirit might be placated and its malignant influence nullified. So long as the practitioner accepted supernatural agencies as the sole cause of disease there could be no advance in the theoretical basis of medical practice.

Lack of a rational theory does not imply that all forms of treatment were useless or that no advance could be made in practical methods. Treatment of disease has never entirely depended upon orthodox theory. Folk medicine owes nothing to scientific thinking, but derives from casual observation that certain herbs or berries will relieve certain symptoms. The two practices, orthodox and unorthodox, borrowed from one another. The folk-doctor enhanced the potency of his simples by appropriate incantations when gathering or administering them. The orthodox physician reinforced his magic with drugs, sometimes borrowed directly from the folk-doctor but often more complex preparations endowed with supernatural qualities. The remedial custom of 'eating the god' which started as ritual cannibalism, the consuming of a sanctified human to absorb divine power, developed into the beginnings of a pharmacopoeia. A symbolic animal or plant took the place of human sacrifice and was eaten to ward off or to undo the ill effect of divine displeasure. The usage persisted long after the underlying tradition had been forgotten. Recognizable traces are to be found in most present-day religions, including the Communion Service of the Anglican Church. Sacrificial meats, the burnt flesh and viscera of animals, blood and excreta, ash cakes of fruits or plants, all played a large part in the early treatment of disease. Just as vestiges of a pagan rite were accepted by the Christian Church, so these traditional remedies remained as part of the orthodox pharmacopoeia until the eighteenth century, although the original source had been forgotten. In a similar manner, the most ancient of surgical operations, trepanning of the skull, is thought to have been based both upon folk observation and orthodox theory. The former suggested that a pressure headache resulting from injury might be relieved by making an aperture in the rigid skull. The second made an opening in the skull to permit egress of an evil spirit which caused the headache. It is thus easy to understand that, from the earliest times until less than two centuries ago, alterations in theory often made little difference to practical treatment.

Most treatment was only effective because the patient had faith in both drug and doctor. Faith healing can work miracles even in our own scientific age. There are miraculous cures today just as there were miraculous cures in ancient Egypt or the early Christian era. The only difference is that the miracle is explicable. We now know that the miracle will succeed when there is no somatic (physical) cause of disease; it will fail if there is a somatic cause. Nor must we fall into the error that a patient who imagines he is ill is not ill. He is ill and can reproduce the symptoms of illness. Such a patient will respond to treatment by a faith healer or by a modern psychiatrist. The treatment works simply because the patient has faith, whether that faith be in his psychiatrist, his physician, his saint, his god, or his magic herb. Further, the faith healer may achieve a limited success in cases of somatic illness. No illness is purely somatic; the existence of any illness effects a psychological change in the patient and such change is amenable to treatment by suggestion. Somatic disease cannot be cured by suggestion but symptoms may be alleviated. Thus we cannot dismiss ancient medicine as useless and we would be unwise to hold that there can have been no advance in treatment. Even the most nonsensical of invocations and the most nauseating of nostrums could have partially relieved suffering provided only that the patient had faith in their efficacy. As the centuries passed, more useful herbal remedies must have been discovered and the practitioner have become increasingly adept in methods of winning the confidence of his patient.

Both theory and practice of medicine have been developed by all civilizations, but the Western world has been more profoundly and more directly influenced by the philosopher-physicians of Greece than by the methods of other nations. The ancient Greeks of the Ionian cities were at one with all primitive races in regarding disease as of supernatural origin.

Bodily illness was a contamination cast upon the soul by infernal gods and spirits in a temporary mood of anger. The orthodox physician sought to avert disease by ritual sacrifice to the gods. In time of sickness he tried to abort illness by rites of propitiation and atonement. If these failed, he endeavoured to expel disease by purification of the individual or of the crowd, in the latter case by sacrifice. Contact with Egypt through Phoenician navigators and possibly with China by the ancient Silk Road probably resulted in some mingling of the medical lore of these older civilizations and may have been the reason for the renunciation of a purely animist or supernatural concept of the universe which became apparent about 600 BC.

The doctrine of four indivisible elements, ascribed to Thales of Miletus who lived 639—544 BC, proposed that all natural substances are compounded of earth, air, fire, and water in varying proportions. About 400 BC Empedocles of Sicily incorporated this doctrine into the philosophy of medicine. To him the four elements formed the basis of all things, including the human body. Health resulted from an equal balance of the four elements, disease from imbalance. We can here observe the first theory of natural causes as opposed to supernatural influence. At about the same time Pythagoras of Samos (580—489 BC) introduced Chaldean number-lore from Egypt. Number-lore to the ancient Greek philosopher was much the same as a computer is to the modern physician. If only he can make it work, it will answer all his questions.

The philosophers used number-lore to evolve the first System of Medicine. Evolution was slow, starting with the theories of Pythagoras, developing through the teaching of Plato and Aristotle in the years 429—322 BC, and reaching a peak under the Arabian alchemists of the thirteenth century AD. The basic idea exerted a profound influence upon medical thought for 1,500 years and so must be briefly described. The early Greek philosophers accepted the four elements and attached a particular significance to the number 4. The nature of the four elements suggested four qualities: dry, cold, hot and moist. The four elements shared these four qualities: hot + dry = fire, hot + moist = air, cold + dry = earth, cold + moist = water. Applied to medicine, the four qualities became four humours, formed as follows: hot + moist = blood, cold + moist = phlegm, hot + dry = yellow bile, cold + dry = black bile. Here indeed is a system of medicine based upon reason, although the reasoning is incorrect. The doctrine of humours persists in common nomenclature. We still speak of a 'bilious attack' when we mean a digestive upset, still use 'phlegmatic' in contradistinction to 'choleric', and often speak of 'good humour' and 'bad humour'. Arabian pharmacists applied the system to remedies which they classified according to degrees or the relative proportions of their several qualities. Their complicated reckoning can be exemplified by two medicaments, commonly prescribed in the thirteenth century although not now used as medicines: Sugar: cold in one degree, warm in two degrees, dry in two degrees, moist in one degree. Or cardamoms which contained one degree of warmth, one-half degree of cold, one degree of dry. Thus we have a classification of diseases and a classification of the drugs employed in treatment.

The Greek philosopher-physician relied to a limited extent upon a knowledge of human anatomy. It is arguable whether he performed dissections, although sometimes accused of dissecting living humans. But he had a unique opportunity of observing surface anatomy and so of correlating internal disease or injury with outward appearances. Greeks were devoted to gymnastics, a term derived from the Greek word for 'naked'. In those sun-drenched lands, athletes customarily performed their exercises entirely unclothed. Thus, as the young athletes ran, jumped, boxed or wrestled, a physician could watch the whole musculature of the body in action and see the relation of muscle to bone and the correct alignment of bones and joints. Since the strenuous sports of these healthy young men produced such injuries as fractures, sprains and dislocations, both gymnast and physician became adept in the treatment of accidents. The physician turned his observations to good account in time of war, when such injuries multiplied. He performed the work of a surgeon but his usefulness was limited because he lacked knowledge of internal disease.

In the year 460 BC Greek medicine was still a philosophy, treatment being unrelated to theory and largely influenced by thaumaturgy. Now dawned the short-lived Golden Age of Greece, the time of Pericles, when Hellenistic art, building and science rose to their peak. About 460 BC there was born the master physician Hippocrates, a man (or perhaps men) usually regarded as the true father of Western European medicine. He is so important in our story that we must consider him again in a later chapter. Here we will confine ourselves to his influence upon medical thought.

It is in fact impossible to assess the influence of Hippocrates during his lifetime, for the simple reason that we do not know how much, if any, of his attributed writings are genuine. There is no existing document bearing his signature or mark and no contemporary record of his work. The oldest known manuscript (in the Vatican library) dates from the tenth century AD and is a compilation from earlier texts. Other versions are of the eleventh and twelfth centuries. Generations of scholars have compared these and other early versions and, by a process of exclusion, have succeeded in reconstructing something which probably resembles the original works of the fifth century BC. A number of passages have been generalized or abbreviated to become proverbs, although their genesis is often forgotten. The well known 'Ars longa, vita brevis' is a Latin form of the opening words of the first Aphorism 'Life is short and the Art long; the occasion fleeting; experience fallacious, and judgement difficult. The physician must not only be prepared to do what is right himself, but also to make the patient, the attendants, and externals co-operate.'

During his traditional lifetime of 90 or 100 years, Hippocrates performed three major services. First, he dissociated medicine from philosophy, transforming the theory into a science in its own right. Second, he rid orthodox medicine of the encumbering priest by refusing to accept supernatural causes or magic remedies. Third, he collected and digested a vast quantity of known facts about disease. He systematized a loose, almost random, collection of theories and observations into a science.

Hippocrates accepted the doctrine of the four humours but combined it with a practical knowledge of anatomy and of disease to form a true humoral pathology. Thus he turned what had previously been pure theory into an applied science. He classed diseases as acute, chronic, endemic and epidemic, a classification which remains good today. Hippocrates was only human and fell into many errors, both in practice and in theory. Perhaps the longest lived and most disastrous is his theory of coction, the supposed process of wound healing in which digestion of the tissues and production of laudable pus is regarded as an essential stage.

Hippocrates was certainly no mere theorist. He is rightly regarded as the founder of bedside medicine. To him the patient was all important. He entirely discarded all vestiges of the ancient idea of demoniac possession, of good spirits warring against bad. He even held that epilepsy 'the Sacred Disease' had a natural although unknown cause.

> It appears to me to be nowise more divine nor more sacred than other diseases, but has a natural cause from which it originates like other infections. Men regard its nature and cause as divine from ignorance and wonder, because it is not at all like other diseases. And this notion of divinity is kept up by their inability to comprehend it, and the simplicity of the mode by which it is cured, for men are freed from it by purifications and incantations.

When we remember that a true epileptic convulsion will cease spontaneously and that 'epilepsy' covered a number of psychiatric disorders, we can understand from the above passage that Hippocrates not only dismissed a supernatural cause but also acknowledged the efficacy of faith healing.

To Hippocrates, somatic disease was an internal battle between morbid matter, a concrete cause, and the natural self-healing power of the body. He would eagerly have accepted the modern theory of bacteria and phagocytes or 'resistance'. Since he accepted the doctrine of humours, his treatment centred upon helping the patient to react against imbalance and so to promote that healthy balance in which natural self-healing would defeat or rid the body of morbid matter. The orthodox pharmacopoeia played little part in his treatment but he believed in the value of some herbs, given in the form of infusions or tisanes. His name became associated with these herbal teas, often referred to as 'Hippocras' until the eighteenth century, although the term was also applied to spiced wine. Hippocrates advocated blood-letting but, for the rest, depended upon the 'regimen', a life of fresh air, controlled exercise, massage and hydrotherapy, assisted by a liberal diet of suitable foods. His system proved successful as is shown by his case-notes which are the first reliable descriptions of patients and their diseases. Hippocrates did not hesitate to report his failures and his notes thus differ from earlier records which are nothing more than votive tablets expressing thanks for a miracle. He tersely describes a fatal case of intestinal obstruction or perhaps acute appendicitis as follows:

> The woman who lodged at the house of Tisamenus had a trouble-some attack of iliac passion: much vomiting: could not keep her drink: pains about the hypochondria, and pains also in the lower part of the belly; constant colic; not thirsty; became hot; extremities cold throughout, with nausea and insomnia; urine scanty and thin; faeces undigested, thin, scanty. Nothing could do her any good. She died.

There are some who hold that Hippocrates was born before his time but it is equally logical to suggest that he arrived at the right moment. He took a volume of already acquired knowledge, purged it of many faults, and reformed it into something far more useful than anything that had previously existed. To early nineteenth-century historians, men like Emile Littré and Francis Adams who translated his works, Hippocrates appeared the greatest physician of all time, one who stood by himself. They tended to disregard the historical evidence that his work was not continued, that, so far from progress, there followed a period of regression. The Golden Age came to a tragic end. The Peloponnesian War, an internecine struggle between the two main Hellenic powers of Athens and Sparta, began in 431 BC. In 430 BC a disastrous pestilence struck Athens, destroying any chance of a quick victory. The war dragged on for twenty-seven years, ending with the total defeat of Athens in 404 BC.

During the century after Hippocrates' death, medical thinking did not follow the clear path opened up by him. He was not only open-minded and receptive of new ideas but had the experimental approach. His successors laid more stress upon dogma than upon investigation; hence the name 'Dogmatists' by which they are known. The dogmatists had inherited a practical science but did little to develop it. More interested in theory, they refused to see medicine as a coherent whole but rigidly differentiated between five subjects: *physiology* implying normal function; *aetiology* or the philosophy of causes; *symptomatology*, which broadly meant the appearance of disease; *hygiene* or the principles of health; *therapeutics* or methods of treatment. The Empiricists, coeval with the dogmatists, based their practice on observation and not upon theory. Following the tradition of folk-doctors, empiricists retained only the divisions of symptomatology and therapeutics, subdividing the latter into surgery, dietetics and pharmacology.

This rather sterile century produced one of the greatest works of all time and one which exerted a profound influence upon medical thought for almost 2,000 years. Aristotle, born about 384 BC was a successor to Plato (429–347 BC). Plato had produced some very extraordinary ideas on natural science. Aristotle, a far better natural historian than Plato, travelled widely in Asia Minor and described about 500 different species of animal. He dissected animals but not the human, applying his findings to both animal and human anatomy. He propounded a Theory of Evolution, the Ladder of Nature, on the lowest rung of which stood inanimate matter, with man on the topmost and plants, insects, reptiles and mammals at intermediate stations. He regarded a living object as inanimate matter imbued with soul, a doctrine accepted in modified forms until the present day. Aristotle's philosophy of medicine depended upon the four elements, qualities and humours. To these he added four temperaments, sanguine, phlegmatic, choleric and melancholic. Aristotle's work was in some measure completed by his pupil Theophrastus, who did for botany what Aristotle had done for the animal kingdom. Theophrastus listed all known medical herbs, assigning to each its property. Although not the earliest Greek herbal, his was the most exact and most complete. Aristotle and Theophrastus created the science of biology. After them, biology ceased to be studied as a science in its own right but for centuries formed part of the philosophy of medicine.

Hellenic power had waned by the time of Theophrastus (c. 300 BC) and Greek learning became dispersed among a number of Mediterranean centres. The chief of these was Alexandria where, under the Greek Ptolemaic dynasty, a flourishing but short lived 'school' of medicine was established. Here Herophilus of Chalcedon, the first man certainly known to have dissected the human body in public, made a number of discoveries chiefly concerning the nervous system. He dismissed earlier teaching that the heart is the centre of intelligence and assigned that function to the brain. His near contemporary Erasistratus is generally regarded as the first true physiologist. He observed that every organ is served by an artery, vein and nerve, which divide and subdivide until invisible to the naked eye. He thought the purpose of these vessels was to provide nourishment: blood through the veins, air through the arteries, and a vital spirit or pneuma through the nerves. His error in regard to arterial function was to be repeated by many later workers, simply because the arteries are empty of blood in the cadaver. Medicine seems to have stagnated at Alexandria about 200 BC, although the 'school' remained famous for its teaching of mathematics and allied subjects.

The independence of Greece virtually ended with the massacre of Corinth in 146 BC, and the territories of the Achaean League came under the dominion of Rome. According to the elder Pliny, the grave and resolute citizens of republican Rome 'had no need of physicians'. They possessed an immense collection of household gods, so numerous that it has been said there was a god for every bodily function and for every known symptom of disease. They had also collected an extensive domestic pharmacopoeia of herbs. The head of the household acted as physician, calling upon the appropriate god and administering the appropriate herb. Failure to cure was easily explicable. The wrong herb had been used or the wrong god invoked.

A few Greeks from the province of Magna Graecia (lower Italy and Eastern Sicily) practised as physicians in Rome. They were objects of suspicion and contempt because the citizens held that they charged fees for treating their patients with barbaric cruelty. The first known Greek physician of Rome, Archagathus, acquired the soubriquet 'Carnifex' because of his lust for surgery. Physicians came from the Greek mainland to Rome in increasing numbers after the destruction of Corinth. Although regarded as slaves, their superior knowledge began to command some respect. Credit for this reversal of opinion is given to Asclepiades who worked in Rome about 100 BC. The name suggests that this may not have been an individual but a family or small company of Greek physicians and there were certainly 'followers of Asclepiades' who maintained the practice for a number of years. They dismissed the Hippocratic teaching of the body's natural healing power and demanded more active measures. Nor did they accept that disease is caused by imbalance of the humours. Instead, they introduced the interesting theory of *'strictum et laxum'*, which has been revived from time to time under various names. Broadly speaking, the theory held that disease was caused by either excess or insufficiency of stimulation.

This was a new theory to be followed by so many more that Graeco-Roman medicine has been aptly described as a 'welter of theorizing'. We have already mentioned that the Alexandrian physician Erasistratus held that a vital principle 'pneuma' was carried by the nerves. The doctrine of pneuma preceded Erasistratus and came to be widely accepted during the 200 years 100 BC to AD 100. As 'pneumatism', a practice based upon the theory, it strongly influenced later medicine. Pneuma is difficult to comprehend and still more difficult to explain in a few words. The theory really attempted to correlate a supernatural *origin* of disease with a natural *cause*. Pneuma cannot be defined in present-day terms. It was not natural air nor a supernatural spirit, but more in the nature of an all-pervading ether or principle. Every phenomenon of life was associated with this principle. It underwent changes in the body, forming a 'vital pneuma' in the heart and an 'animal pneuma' in the brain. At the moment of death the body surrendered its share of pneuma which mingled with the universal supply.

Three men of the first century AD influenced later development, not because of their discoveries but through their writings. The first, Dioscorides, a Greek surgeon in the army of Nero, employed his spare time studying plants and is the 'Roman' equivalent of the 'Greek' Theophrastus. Less of a botanist and more of a pharmacologist, he is usually regarded as the originator of the *materia medica*. Dioscorides described over 600 medicinal plants, of which 149 were known to Hippocrates; some ninety are still to be found in the pharmacopoeia, although usually in the form of an active principle rather than the herb itself. It is almost impossible to overrate the influence of his work which formed the basis of herbal therapy for at least 1,600 years. Early books on medical botany are little more than commentaries upon his original treatise.

Celsus, who was probably born about the year AD 13, was not a Greek but a Roman of noble birth who wrote a great encyclopaedia or perhaps translated an earlier, unknown, text into Latin. Celsus covered a very wide field; it is probable that his writings were intended as a book of household management from which the master could distribute advice. We learn from Celsus that the Romans were quite advanced in their practice of surgery, which is not surprising if we recall the Hippocratic dictum 'War is the only proper school for the surgeon'. The writings of Celsus probably affected domestic medicine for a number of years and are now of great historical interest. He had no direct influence upon mediaeval medicine; only four references to his works have been discovered in mediaeval commentaries. His *De Re Medicina* was apparently unknown until Pope Nicholas V discovered a manuscript during the first half of the fifteenth century. This was one of the first medical books to be printed (Florence, 1478) and passed through a number of editions.

Lastly we come to Galen, the brilliant physician whose teaching dominated medicine for over 1,200 years. He was a Greek, born at Pergamon in Asia Minor in AD 131, who settled in Rome about the year 160 and acquired a reputation which gained him the title 'Clarissimus'. He was the most prolific of ancient medical writers. According to legend, Galen's works started as a brief treatise written in 165. This was accidentally destroyed in a fire. He then rewrote his text on a much larger scale, finishing the series of books in 177. A large number of these manuscripts were lost in another fire in 192. Nothing daunted, Galen reconstructed and enlarged his work into a vast encyclopaedia which was 'published' at some time between 192 and his death in 201. Complete and original texts are said to have been available in the Near East as late as the ninth century, but all surviving manuscripts in Western Europe derive from a single incomplete and mutilated example. The full text, derived from the Near East, was not in fact known in the West until the nineteenth century.

Much of Galen's work is a compilation of older knowledge, but he was no mere commentator. He performed a considerable amount of original work in anatomy and experimental physiology. Galen did not dissect or experiment upon the human body. He used animals—apes or pigs—and applied his findings to man. Thus he fell into errors which were perpetuated for centuries. He came to the conclusion that blood, formed in the liver, passed through the vessels by an ebb-and-flow movement. This mistaken idea was not fully disproved until the seventeenth century.

Galen accepted both the doctrines of humours and pneuma. He retained the Hippocratic theory of coction, thus perpetuating the fallacy that suppuration (laudable pus) is an essential stage of wound healing. He closely followed the teaching of Hippocrates in his methods of treatment but added a great number of herbal remedies which were still spoken of as 'galenicals' in the nineteenth century. He did not use herbs as 'simples', that is as single entities, but in complex mixtures. For this reason he has sometimes been called the first polypharmacist. Galen was dogmatic in all his writings, regarding himself as infallible. He produced an explanation for every one of his statements, but the majority of his 'explanations' depended upon theory unsupported by proof.

Galen's supreme service to medicine lies in his writings, through which Greek theory and practice were transmitted to the mediaeval world.

A lesser man than Hippocrates, he provided the channel through which the teachings of Hippocrates became widely spread. But Galen was regarded as the ultimate authority. His works were copied and recopied, translated and retranslated. No one dared question his findings, no one dared correct the disastrous errors into which he had fallen. This is why we have concentrated here upon his mistakes rather than upon the real advances which he made. The tragedy of Galen is that he, one of the first and greatest of experimentalists, became the dead hand which held back all experiment, all advances, for centuries after his death.

The reason is to be found in the Roman and Christian attitudes towards medicine. The Roman public health service was superb. Water supply, sanitation, inspection of food supplies, cremation of the dead, are some of the measures which made Roman cities more pleasant to live in than the Paris or London of 1,000 years later. Their much vaunted medical service and the state schools which supplied medical officers were less satisfactory. Instituted purely for the needs of the army, the service demanded practical surgeons rather than intellectual physicians. The 'wound doctor' of the Roman army, himself a legionary, approximated more to the *feldsher* of the Imperial Russian regime than to an officer in the RAMC. A system such as this is unlikely to produce critical thinkers and certainly not men of a calibre to challenge the authoritarian Galen.

The first century AD witnessed the gradual emergence of a new philosophy. Jewish or Biblical medicine is notable for insistence upon a high standard of social hygiene. Disease itself was an expression of the wrath of God, only to be countered by moral reform, prayer and sacrifice. After the Dispersion, following the war of AD 66, small Jewish communities established themselves in Roman domains along the Mediterranean seaboard. They brought their philosophy with them. They also brought a long tradition of care for the sick and unfortunate.

The Jews were accompanied by a few adherents to a new faith which had grown up around the teaching and example of Jesus Christ. It is a matter of opinion whether the Christian religion spread so widely and so quickly because it offered new hope in a period of great sickness and mortality. It is no matter of opinion, but undeniable fact, that the ministry of healing was a special function of the early Church. 'He called his twelve disciples together, and gave them power and authority over all devils, and to cure diseases.' (*St Luke* ix. 1.) This authority was transmitted to the hierarchy. The power, derived originally from the Son of God, is passed from generation to generation. The symbolism still remains in the Anglican Church when the attendant bishops crowd around their newly consecrated colleague and touch him with their hands.

Christianity was in part a revolt against the pessimism of pagan materialism as it had developed in the hands of Greek and Roman. The Christian relied upon supernatural aid and so he returned to a supernatural concept of disease. Borrowing the disease-provoking wrath of God from his Jewish predecessors and the healing ministry of Christ from the apostles, he discarded any teaching which insisted on a natural cause or envisaged a human cure. The physician could alleviate but he could not cure; all cures were miraculous. Christianity also borrowed a number of Roman gods, or gods which the Romans had themselves acquired from exotic sources. These were transformed into saints, sometimes with little change of name or function. Thus Febris, the goddess of fever, became Saint Febronia, a lady now regarded as mythical. More interesting is the case of St Sebastian, also now regarded as mythical although he can boast a detailed legend. The god Apollo fired his arrows of disease and therefore had to be placated in times of pestilence. The symbolism of the arrow occurs throughout the Sebastian story. Ordered to be shot to death, he survived to undergo a second martyrdom by flogging in the arena. Early representations depict him as an elderly man, fully clothed. In one such he is turning an arrow aside with his cloak. Later pictures show him as a naked youth of great physical beauty. He has become the patron of epidemic disease and fully identified with the beauteous Apollo. After the Renaissance, a time of plague, one arrow is usually found transfixing the groin, a reminder that bubonic plague commonly causes swelling of the inguinal glands. The Christian invoked his saint just as the Roman invoked his god. Medical theory and much of medical practice had seemingly regressed to the beginning of time.

But the regression was only partial. Christians could accept the doctrine of humours and temperaments because God had created the healthy balance and He alone permitted imbalance. They could also accept the theory of pneuma, translating it from vitalism, the origin of life in a vital principle, to animism, life produced by an immaterial soul or the Spirit of God breathed into inanimate clay. It did not require much ingenuity to weave Greek theories of medicine into the fabric of a belief in an Almighty God who alone could inflict and cure disease. But this is not the whole truth. The orthodox priest-physician of ancient times relied upon gods and incantations but needed a pharmacopoeia. The early Christian Church tended to frown upon scientific theories but placed no ban upon learning. Knowledge had been extended by scientists and mathematicians, by anatomists and natural historians. The Christian physician demanded a compendium of the sciences and he found this in the writings of Galen. It is thus understandable that Galen, once accepted, would in time be regarded as the sole authority.

While Rome crumbled to its fall, Christianity began to develop into an organized society. The steady flame of learning died in Western Europe, leaving only small flickering lights where the tiny Christian communities lived insecurely, surrounded by hostile and pagan tribes. We speak of the next 600 years as the age of Monastic Medicine and, as may be readily understood, we know very little of it. The great majority of Europeans depended upon a kind of magic folk-medicine, the ancient blend of herbs and spells to be found in Anglo-Saxon leech books. Here is an example from *Lacnunga*, a sort of physician's common-place book. The manuscript from which it is taken dates from about AD 1000, but contains much that has been copied from earlier works. The Holy Salve (a dressing for wounds) is to be made from sixty named herbs, the largest proportion to be of lovage, alexanders, parsley and groundsel. These are to be mixed with butter

> And thus shall the butter be made for the holy salve: Let the butter be churned from a cow of all one colour, so that she be all red or all white without markings; and if thou have not butter enough, wash other butter very clean and mix with it. And shred up all the plants together very small; and hallow water with font-hallowing; and put a bowl of it in the butter. Then take a stick and make four prongs to it. Write on the face of the prongs these holy names: Matthew, Mark, Luke, John. Then stir the butter with the stick, the whole vessel. Do thou sing over it these psalms: 'Beati Immaculati', each section thrice over it, and 'Gloria in Excelsis Deo' and 'Credo in Deum Patrem' and recite litanies over it, that is, the names of the saints and 'Deus Meus et Pater' and 'In Principio' and let this charm be sung over it: 'Acre Arcre Arnem Nona Aernem Beooora Aernem: Nidren Arcun Cunao Ele Harassan Fidine.' Sing this nine times, and put thy spittle on the plants and blow on them and lay them by the bowl and afterwards let a mass-priest hallow them. Let him sing these prayers over them: 'Holy Lord, Omnipotent Father, Eternal God: by the laying on of my hands may the enemy, the Devil, depart from the hairs, from the head, from the eyes, from the nose, from the lips, from the tongue, from the undertongue, from the neck, from the breast, from the feet, from the heels, from the whole framework of his members, so that the Devil may have no power over him, neither in his speech nor in his silence, neither in his sleeping nor in his waking, neither by day nor by night, neither in resting nor in running, neither in seeing nor in smiling, neither in writing nor in reading: So be it in the Name of the Lord Jesus Christ, Who redeemed us with His Holy Blood, Who liveth with the Father and reigneth God, world without end. Amen.

Professor J. H. G. Grattan and Professor Charles Singer say of this excerpt (which is taken from their book *Anglo-Saxon Magic and Medicine*, London, Oxford University Press, 1952) 'The juxtaposition of (a) the gibberish chant, (b) the use of spittle, (c) the blowing on the wound, and (d) the Christian chant of the priest, is impressive as a summary of Anglo-Saxon magic.' Yet even these leech books contain recognizable fragments of Hippocratic teaching, and we know that the heritage of Greek medicine was not entirely lost. Monastic scribes copied and circulated Galenic texts as well as religious works. When a stable society emerged from the chaos, Western European practice was still in a sufficiently flourishing state to absorb the more virile medicine of the Middle East.

Rome annexed Asia Minor in the first century BC. Four hundred years later Constantine the Great founded his capital of Byzantium and this, the Eastern Empire or Second Rome, survived as a Christian centre until taken by Mohammed II in 1453. The practice of medicine fell entirely into the hands of priests who slavishly conformed to ancient teaching. We should know little of Byzantine medicine but for the writings of Oribasius, Aëtius of Amida, Alexander of Tralles (brother of the architect of St Sophia) and Paul of Aegina. These men were compilers rather than original thinkers. Paul frankly admitted that Galen and his predecessors had said everything worth while on the subject and that he was a mere scribe. Byzantium added little or nothing to medical knowledge but preserved some of the culture and many of the texts of Greece. The manuscripts were not originals but were earlier and less corrupt copies than those available in Western Europe. The medical scholar Sir Clifford Allbutt wrote 'The chief monuments of learning were stored in Byzantium until Western Europe was fit to take care of them.'

In 431 the Patriarch of Constantinople, Nestorius, decided that the Virgin Mary should be styled Mother of Christ and not Mother of God. This theological quibble is the starting point of Arabian medicine. Banished for heresy, Nestorius fled with a small band of supporters to Edessa (Urfa) in Mesopotamia. Persecuted again in 489, the Nestorian Christians moved further east and settled at the lost town of Jundi-shapur. They occupied part of the next two centuries with the translation of Greek texts into Syriac and Arabic. These included some of Hippocrates, Dioscorides and Galen, older versions probably derived from Alexandria. In the seventh century the Moslem Empire engulfed Persia which now contained a number of Nestorian communities. Moslems encouraged science and tolerated Christian physicians; thus several Nestorians rose to quite high positions. One of them, Gabriel, became physician to the court of Haroun al Raschid. Two more, both Persians by birth, added to medical literature. Rhazes (Abu Becr Mohammed Ibn Zacariya Ar-Razi) wrote a great number of books about 900 AD including a volume on smallpox and measles which is still regarded as a classic. The position of the second, Avicenna (Abu Ali al Hussein ibn Abdallah ibn Sina born in 980) is more difficult to assess. Described by some authorities as 'a professional scribbler' and by others as 'the summit of excellence in Arabian medicine', his great work *The Canon of Medicine* was a text book in common use as late as 1650. But he misinterpreted much of the good sense in Galen's writings while adopting his dogmatic style. Perhaps his long authority depends more upon self-confidence than upon merit.

The Moslem Empire spread west into Southern Spain. Here important medical centres were established, particularly that of Cordova. The Western Caliphate produced good doctors such as Avenzoar, died in 1162, who had the courage to question the authority of Galen, and the Jew Moses ben Maimon, known as Maimonides, who was persecuted for his faith, became court physician to Saladin, and is thought to have been taken by Sir Walter Scott as the original of El Hakim in *Talisman*. Maimonides opposed all forms of magic and instituted a real search for the cause of disease. He wrote a small synopsis of Galen's works, a valuable book for the ordinary physician who had little time to plough through a mass of manuscripts. Albucasis or Abulkasim, born near Cordova in 1013, produced valuable treatises on surgery, giving detailed descriptions of the treatment of wounds and methods of performing amputations and other operations such as lithotomy.

The Arabian physicians had a better knowledge of Greek medicine than the physicians of Western Europe because they possessed more perfect texts of Galen. But they did not advance theory to any great extent, contenting themselves with discussion as to the exact meaning of passages in the old manuscripts. The main usefulness of Arabian medicine lay in an important practical contribution to the pharmacopoeias and to para-medical science. Alchemy derived from herbal lore and is the ancestor of chemistry. The underlying philosophy supposed a 'soul' of the world and 'spirits' of all natural things. Alchemists sought to extract the spirit from the substance. They held metals to be generated in the bowels of the earth and searched for the germinal agent. Here is the basis of the alchemist's quest for a means of producing gold. He did not so much seek to transmute base metals as to find the agent responsible for producing natural gold in the earth. Hand in hand with this primary enquiry went a search for potable gold, held to be the polyvalent medicine or elixir of life which would renew youth by total cure of all disease. Experiments on a large scale produced many incidental and valuable discoveries. By the end of the thirteenth century Arabian pharmacopoeias listed over 1,400 preparations. The most influential, *Grabadin* or the apothecary's manual, was compiled by Mesuë (probably a pseudonym) in the eleventh century. The Arabian original has never been found but it became the most popular of European pharmacopoeias in a Latin translation and was one of the earlier medical books to be printed.

The ninth century saw a limited fusion of Monastic and Arabian medicine in the school of Salerno, which we shall consider at greater length in another chapter. Graduates of the school spread throughout Western Europe, even into Britain. They brought with them some knowledge of Arabian medicine. The term 'Arabian medicine' does not refer to nationality but to the language used by the doctors who were often Jews and Christians. As Moslem power waned, the Latin-speaking priestly and upper classes started to move into Southern Spain and developed a tri-lingual culture. Adventurous spirits, already knowing something of Arabian medicine from Salernitan doctors, began to search out the sources of their knowledge in the old Moslem centres of Southern Europe. They translated Arabic manuscripts into Latin with the aid of Jews and Mahommedans. These Arabic manuscripts were themselves translations of Greek texts, often via Syriac, and abounded in errors, additions and emendations. We cannot wonder if the new Latin versions bore little resemblance to the originals.

Confusion was to be worse confounded. Medical philosophy in Northern and Western Europe, now firmly in the hands of the Church, had become an educational discipline almost totally divorced from the bedside. The new texts were eagerly studied and then treated in a manner similar to that of the Arabian scholars. Argument and counter-argument, splitting of hairs, the disputed meaning of a word took the place of rational discussion and practical investigation. This was the golden age of the scholiast and dialectician. Ecclesiastical authority stifled creative thought and discouraged experiment. Human anatomy remained the anatomy of ape and pig as described by Galen. It is widely held that the Church actually forbade dissection, a misreading of a Bull promulgated by Boniface VIII which prohibited boiling and dismembering the corpses of dead crusaders in order to return their bones for burial. But the Church, believing in physical resurrection, frowned upon dissection and the frown of the Church could be as dangerous as its ban. A few brave men defied opinion. Roger Bacon was certainly an experimental scientist although he produced little new. But he aroused the mistrust of his Franciscan superiors who condemned him to prison. Mondino de Luzzi (Mundinus) dissected human bodies in the period 1275—90. His findings were not published until the fifteenth century and even he recorded 'we might understand the temporal bone better if it were cleaned by boiling but this is sinful'.

The fourteenth century witnessed an increasing revolt against repression by Holy Church. Partly this was due to the scandal of rival Popes at Rome and Avignon. But the terrible conditions of life which developed in the second half of the century provided a greater stimulus. Sickness and mortality on an unprecedented scale, famine and war, not only weakened the Church by loss of manpower and revenue, but caused thinking men to question the authority by which churchmen held power over their bodies and their souls. In the limited sphere of medicine, loss of confidence in the clerical physician caused a proliferation of quack doctors and bizarre theories. The pseudo-science of astrology rose to its highest peak in the late fourteenth and fifteenth centuries. An important part of Arabian medicine and of Chaldean philosophy, astrology derived from the observation that tides are influenced by phases of the moon. The immoveable Earth was regarded as the centre of a finite universe of celestial bodies moving in ordered progress from one part of the firmament to another. Since the moon exerted so great an influence upon the seas, it was reasonable to suppose that all heavenly bodies influenced the earth and its inhabitants to a greater or lesser degree. Physician-astrologers assigned the seven planets to the seven major bodily organs, the seven days of the week, and the seven metals, and so worked out a system of specific treatment. They also used astrology as a means of prognosis which called for an involved calculation of the various planets' position at the time of the patient's birth and at the commencement of his illness. A curious offshoot of astrology is known as uroscopy or water casting, described by a later and more outspoken generation as 'piss-prophecy'. The art derived from the very ancient rite of casting the auspices coupled with an Arabian belief that the sex of an unborn child can be determined by examination of the mother's urine. When shorn of astrological nonsense, uroscopy became of real use as a diagnostic aid, since the presence of blood, bile, or a heavy sediment in the urine would indicate the nature of an ailment. The method remained a popular one and may be regarded as the ancestor of biochemistry.

The voyages of discovery pioneered by Prince Henry the Navigator and the invention of printing belong to the fifteenth century. The first widened the horizon of the European and the second widened his reading. In 1453 came the fall of Byzantium when a flood of refugees poured into Italy bringing with them many of the priceless manuscripts with which the city had been stored. Latin was the language of the mediaeval period. Now the Latin texts were flung aside and the scholar turned to Greek. Physicians at last had the opportunity of examining older and relatively uncorrupt texts of Hippocrates and Galen, of Dioscorides and Aristotle. They came to their work with new, enquiring minds and they discovered how filled with errors, interpolations and misunderstandings were the standard text books of their predecessors. An example of these new men is the physician-priest Thomas Linacre who travelled from England to Italy, and is said to have been the first Englishman to understand Aristotle and Galen in their Greek forms. He restored Galen's authority by an accurate translation of several Greek manuscripts back into Latin.

It is sometimes claimed for Linacre that he was the first British apostle of the European Renaissance. The Renaissance was not simply a revival of classical learning and art, but a new freedom of thought, a questioning of traditional ideas. Hardly had the teachings of the ancients been restored to their purity when men started to object that the teaching was false. The age of the scholiast passed and the age of the experimentalist opened. Artists such as Michelangelo, Raphael, and Dürer began to study the human body and found that an accurate knowledge of anatomy is essential when representing a figure in action. They all dissected the cadaver and made discoveries. The most brilliant of these Renaissance artists, Leonardo da Vinci, was the first man to question the accuracy of Galen's anatomy. He planned a text book in collaboration with a medical teacher, Marcantonio della Torre, but the project was never finished.

The first great anatomical treatise, *De Humanis Corporis Fabrica* by Andreas Vesalius appeared in 1543. About nine years before this date, Vesalius studied medicine in Paris under Jacques Dubois, a man in his late fifties. Dubois taught from a Galenic text with such fidelity that, if he found any structure not conforming to Galen's description, he maintained that the human body must have changed since the first century AD. The strange point is that Dubois, better known as Sylvius, was a good anatomist who made a number of discoveries. Although he described his famous pupil as a madman, Dubois probably inspired Vesalius. Appointed prosector and professor at Padua when still a young man, Vesalius encountered such hostility on the publication of his great work that he resigned the chair in disgust. His *Fabrica* is now recognized as the boundary between ancient and modern anatomy.

Reawakened interest in anatomy stimulated advances in surgery, of which art it is the science. Galen described surgery as 'only a means of treatment', implying inferiority of the surgeon to the physician. Arabian commentators went further; they held it unclean and unholy to touch the human body with the hands. Churchmen were forbidden to practise any form of treatment which involved shedding of blood, as laid down at the Council of Tours in 1163 *Ecclesia abhorret a sanguine*. Surgery, which included dentistry and blood-letting, fell largely into the hands of itinerant quacks such as barbers, bath-keepers and sow-gelders. But surgery is at all times needful and especially so in warfare. The Frenchman Ambroise Paré served from 1536 as an army surgeon and ended his military career with the reputation of the foremost surgeon in Europe. He devised artificial limbs, discovered that gunshot wounds are not necessarily poisoned, replaced treatment with boiling oil and cauterization by soothing ointments, and introduced ligation of bleeding vessels in place of searing.

In medical theory, Jean Francois Fernel of Clermont tried to discover the cause of disease by a study of physiology and pathology, publishing a text book on the subject in 1554. A more exciting and controversial figure is his Swiss contemporary Aureolus Theophrastus Bombastus von Hohenheim who, in addition to this resounding name, acquired the pseudonym of Paracelsus. He is variously described as a genius, a drunkard, and a sufferer from one of the end results of syphilis, general paralysis of the insane. There is no reason why he should not have been all three. Appointed professor of medicine at Basel in 1527, his first act was to burn publicly the works of Galen and Avicenna. Paracelsus recognized five causes of disease: cosmic agencies, pathological poisons, predisposition, psychic and divine intervention. He had faith in alchemy and astrology and it is for this reason that he introduced a number of metallic salts into the pharmacopoeia. The kind of change which he effected can be exemplified by his treatment of lung infections. Conservative physicians used an old fashioned magical remedy, a decoction of hoglice. Paracelsus advised inhalation of the fumes of burning sulphur. His treatment was probably no more effective but at least depended upon reason and not upon superstition. Perhaps his most serious contribution to medical science was his observation that certain diseases are associated with mining and that cretinism and goitre are coincident in some Alpine areas. But the real importance of Paracelsus does not lie in his opinions or suggestions. He influenced both his contemporaries and his successors by a rebellion against accepted ideas.

The Reformation further weakened the power of the Church, virtually destroying its temporal authority in England and parts of the European continent. Belief in supernatural causes and intervention still remained. Paré's often quoted dictum 'I dressed the patient but God healed him' is not only an unusual example of surgical humility but an acknowledgement of the divine prerogative. Heretical ideas remained dangerous. In 1553 Michael Servetus, a Spaniard who had studied medicine in France, published *Christianismi Restitutio*, a book in which he propounded the theory of a lesser or pulmonary circulation of the blood, partially contradicting the ebb-and-flow movement described by Galen. A few months later, when Servetus was in Geneva, the book came to the attention of the Protestant leader John Calvin who condemned the unfortunate author to be burned alive on 27 October 1553. His work contained other heresies and he is a religious rather than a medical martyr, although often claimed as the latter.

A new approach to science developed largely through the work of Francis Bacon in England and René Descartes in Holland. Bacon urged philosophers to abandon old methods and to replace them by inductive reasoning based on experience. Descartes held that thought is the essence of existence: 'I think, therefore I am.' He considered the body as a machine. Animals were automata because they did not possess minds or souls. Man, although also a machine, possessed a mind which activated his body at will. This combination of a 'thinking machine' and 'inductive reasoning' is the foundation of the experimental approach, conclusions reached by logical thought based upon observation. A notable exponent of inductive reasoning is William Harvey, who discovered the circulation of the blood and finally disproved Galen's ebb-and-flow theory. Harvey's *Exercitatio Anatomica de Motu Cordis et Sanguinis in Animalibus* (1628) is not only a medical classic but the first true text book of experimental physiology. His 'circulation of the blood' was no mere speculation, but positive fact proved by rational observation and experiment.

Harvey did not use a microscope and so was unable to see how blood passed from the arterioles to the venules. Primitive microscopes, no better than single magnifying lenses, were probably known in the thirteenth century AD. In 1609 a Dutch spectacle maker, Zacharius Jansen, placed two lenses in a tube. Athanasius Kircher of Würzburg examined the blood of plague victims through an instrument of this kind and described 'masses of small worms' which he thought to be the cause of plague. They were probably clumps of red blood corpuscles. An Italian, Marcello Malpighi, discovered the existence of the capillary network in 1660. His finding was confirmed and shown to be an anastomosis between arterioles and venules by Anton van Leeuwenhoek of Delft, using an improved microscope of his own design.

The question of *how* the blood circulates had now been answered. *Why* the blood circulates is a different problem. Harvey had no definite views on the subject. General opinion held that it had something to do with body temperature, blood being warmed by the heart and cooled in the lungs. Four young Oxford scientists supplied the correct answer. Robert Boyle in 1660, having devised an air-pump, showed that neither a flame nor a mouse could exist when the container was exhausted. Air is therefore an essential of combustion and of life. Robert Hooke demonstrated in 1667 that artificial respiration can keep an animal alive, thus proving that lung movement is essential *only* to take in and expel air. Two years later Richard Lower injected dark venous blood into lungs and insufflated them with air, concluding that the bright red change in the colour of the blood is due to absorption of air as it passes through the lungs. Finally John Mayow showed that the 'fire-air' part of ordinary air changed the colour of dark venous blood to bright red. He extracted his 'fire-air' from potassium nitrate and had thus used oxygen. By 1670 the basic elements of circulatory and respiratory physiology had been established.

The seventeenth century saw the foundation of a number of

societies destined to exercise a profound influence upon the development of science and medicine. The Accademia dei Lincei at Rome is the earliest, commencing work in 1603. In 1645 a small group formed the 'invisible college' which met at Gresham College, London. A few years later the Oxford scientists began to meet regularly for discussion. In 1662 these two associations fused into one, dedicated to the improvement of natural science, to become the Royal Society of London. Their influential journal *Philosophical Transactions* started publication two years later. The equally influential Academie des Sciences in Paris was founded under the patronage of Louis XIV in 1666.

At the end of the seventeenth century Isaac Newton established a new theory of the universe and a new approach to natural science which finally ended the ancient authority of Aristotle, Galen, and the mediaeval philosophers. Newton and the great botanist Carl Linné (Linnaeus) introduced classification and orderly thinking into natural science. The next 100 years was a time of great physicians, fine teachers such as Hermann Boerhaave of Leyden and William Cullen of Glasgow and Edinburgh among many others, who made no revolutionary discoveries but who translated theory into bedside medicine. Theories of disease abounded. Animism, the blending of body and soul, was advocated by G. E. Stahl of Halle, and vitalism, a dominant force neither body nor soul, by Joseph Barthez of Montpellier. Friedrich Hoffman reverted to something resembling pneuma which maintained the body in equilibrium. This was not unlike the ancient doctrine of *'strictum et laxum'* and resembles the Brunonian System taught by John Brown, a pupil of Cullen. He divided all diseases into sthenic and asthenic, diseases of increased and diminished sensibility. His theory aroused intense partisanship throughout Europe for a quarter of a century. In 1802 a battle between Brunonian and anti-Brunonian students at Gottingen lasted two days until ended by the intervention of a troop of cavalry.

The most revolutionary of all eighteenth century discoveries is the first preparation of carbon dioxide gas by Joseph Black of Glasgow in 1757. The discovery of carbon dioxide stimulated a new chemistry and new work on the physiology of respiration. It led to the discovery of oxygen by Joseph Priestley in 1774. Antoine Laurent Lavoisier transformed chemistry by discarding the old phlogiston theory and substituting the theory of oxidation. He also showed that the oxygen of inspired air is converted into the carbon dioxide contained in expired air. Twenty year old Humphry Davy was the first to indicate that oxygen is carried in the arterial blood and carbon dioxide in the venous. But the primary importance of Black's discovery lies in the fact that carbon dioxide is impalpable and invisible yet possesses chemical properties. Such a statement is so obvious today as to be not worth making. It was not at all obvious to men of the eighteenth century. The gases helped to condition their minds to the existence of other matter which could not be felt or perceived by unaided human vision.

Carl Linné's botanical system suggested that diseases might be classified in the same way, signs and symptoms playing the part of petals or leaves and occurring in a similar orderly and unvarying manner. Brown had taken a number of diseases and tried to force them into two classes. For centuries medical philosophers had searched for the *cause of disease*. In the eighteenth century they began to look for the *causes of diseases*. Giovanni Battista Morgagni of Padua performed a very great number of autopsies and in 1761, when seventy-nine years old, published a five-volume book in which he correlated postmortem appearances with clinical symptoms. Then came Marie Francois Xavier Bichat of Paris, founder of the science of histology, who held that individual diseases affect individual membranes (tissues) rather than the whole body or the gross bodily organs. He paved the way for the cell theory of Rudolf Virchow which belongs to modern medicine.

The concept of separate diseases rather than 'disease' demanded accurate means of diagnosis. The physician depended, and continued to depend for many years to come, upon his five senses. Even the pulse could not be properly timed until John Floyer introduced a special watch, running for one minute, in 1707. The clinical thermometer came into limited use only at the end of the eighteenth century. Leopold Auenbrugger, a physician of Vienna, was an innkeeper's son who had often rapped casks of wine to ascertain the fluid level. He applied the method to the human chest and so introduced the technique of percussion, which he described in a small book in 1761. The complementary method of auscultation is the contribution of René Theophile Hyacinthe Laennec, physician to the Necker Hospital in Paris. He is supposed to have noticed two children playing with a hollow log, one tapping it and the other listening at the open end. His first stethoscopes (1819) were of paper, rolled into a cylinder. Laennec later made a wooden instrument and described the various sounds he heard with its aid. The names which he coined for these sounds are still in use today.

There is a very old theory that pestilence and wound infections are carried or caused by bad air. The idea is expressed in the term 'malaria'. In 1717 Giovanni Maria Lancisi of Rome published a book *De Noxiis Paludum Effluviis*. Lancisi recognized that mosquitoes played some part, but held malaria to be caused by a poison carried in the air. This 'something in the air' is quite different from 'bad air'. The theory of miasma or pythogenic theory, as understood by physicians and surgeons in the first half of the nineteenth century, depended upon a poisonous effluent, probably a gas from cesspits and sewers, which was borne in the air to an open wound or to the lungs. The miasma caused a disease. Air then conveyed miasma from one patient to another and so produced an epidemic. In the early 1860s Joseph Lister of Glasgow carried the theory one stage further when he told his students that 'the something' carried in the air, the miasma, probably was not a gas or an effluvium but more in the nature of a fine dust resembling pollen. Here is the stepping stone which leads us from ancient to present-day medicine.

2 The care of the sick before 1800

The first known hospitals were temples dedicated to Aesculapius (Asklepios), the son of Apollo, chief god of healing in the Greek pantheon. They sprang up in all parts of the Eastern Mediterranean; remains are still to be seen on the Island of Cos, at Epidauros and Pergamon. The temples were sited in peaceful surroundings, in woods or on mountainsides, close to a source of pure water or a mineral spring. Here the sick came for 'temple sleep' or 'incubation'. The sufferer made prayer and sacrifice, was purified by lustration, a ceremonial washing with water from the spring, and received a preliminary treatment of massage and inunction with oils. He then lay down to sleep in the sanctuary where a priest appeared to him in the guise of the god. A consultation followed if the patient was awake. If he slept, he received advice in a dream, afterwards interpreted by the priest, who then prescribed appropriate treatment. Fortunate patients might be visited by the sacred serpents of Apollo or even by the god himself.

The treatment, if not entirely magical, contained a large element of magic. Incubation has persisted as a method of treating illness from about 1000 BC until the present day, for it is still practised in the Greek Islands. The reason for this long history is to be found in a modification which became apparent during the second century BC. The temples developed into health resorts, not unlike modern spas. Patients no longer stayed for a single night but remained for days or weeks, taking baths, drinking medicinal water, following a strict regimen of diet, controlled exercise and massage. The attendant priests acquired some knowledge of hypnosis which they used both to induce sleep and to suggest alleviation of symptoms. They seem to have been men of common sense, tinctured with humour. Aristides, a hypochondriac, left an account of his treatment at Pergamon. The god ordered him to rub himself all over with mud, to wash in the well, and to run naked three times round the temple. There was a keen frost and a north wind that night. Aristides admitted the treatment had done him good.

Many older medical historians gave credit to the Romans as the founders of the hospital system for care and treatment of the sick. More recent research suggests that Roman medicine was not so advanced as the older school believed. For instance, 'surgical instruments' discovered at

Pompeii are now thought to be ordinary craftsmens' tools. The only civilian hospital known to have existed in the time of the Empire is that on the Island of St Bartholomew in the Tiber. Even this appears to have been more of a refuge for unwanted sick slaves than a hospital in the modern sense. The slaves may have been exposed on the island to avoid the trouble of treating an illness. The place became a haven for sick poor and organized care developed at a much later date. Valetudinaria were certainly established on the frontiers, available both for the army and for civilian officials. It must, however, be questioned whether these were 'hospitals' or rest-houses in which worn-out, dying, and seriously wounded people, unable to defend themselves, might be protected from hostile tribes. Physicians in the larger cities often received patients into their homes but it is likely that such establishments catered only for those who could pay high fees.

In AD 335 pagan temples were closed by decree of Constantine. These included the Asclepieia. Foundation of Christian 'hospitals' immediately followed, perhaps instigated by Constantine's mother, Helena. At first quite small, the hospitals quickly grew in size. In 369 St Basil founded a large establishment at Cappadocia while the plague hospital at Edessa (375) is believed to have had accommodation for over 300 patients. The Byzantine Empire is well- known as a period of hospital foundation and these seem to have been on a large scale. The famous Hôtel Dieu in Paris is believed to date from between 641 and 691, although the first indisputable record is not until 829.

In all aspects of disease the Christian emphasis was upon *care* rather than upon *cure*. We saw in the first chapter that Christianity insisted upon a supernatural cause of disease and would only admit a supernatural cure. Thus the devoted care of sick persons tended to express itself in comfort, support, and alleviation of symptoms rather than in attempts to deal with the underlying disease. Since the object was to help a 'patient' to bear his misfortunes, it followed that a 'hospital' admitted a variety of unfortunates whom we should not class as sick today. Just before the Church foundations were suppressed by the Tudors, a London citizen named Robert Copland described the kinds of people admitted to a hospital. He speaks through the mouth of a gate porter, probably of St Bartholomew's in Smithfield:

> They that be at such mischief
> That for their living can do no labour
> And have no friends to do them succour:
> As old people sick and impotent,
> Poor women in childbed here have easement,
> Weak men sore wounded by great violence
> And sore men eaten with pox and pestilence,
> And honest folk fallen in great poverty
> By mischance or other infirmity;
> Wayfaring men and maimed soldiers
> Have their relief in this poor-house of ours;

And all others which we deem good and plain
Have their lodging here for a night or twain;
Bedrid folks and such as cannot crave
In these places most relief they have,
And if they hap within our place to die
Then are they buried well and honestly.
But not every unsick stubborn knave
For then we should over many have.

Thus a hospital founded for the relief of the sick admitted practically every type of unfortunate except 'stubborn knaves'. For this reason it is quite impossible to determine the exact purpose of the hundreds of hospitals founded in Britain between the introduction of Christianity and the Reformation. The majority were 'places of resort' which is the ancient meaning of the word.

There is a commonly held fallacy that every monastery, priory, and abbey administered a hospital. The mistaken belief has arisen because monastic houses usually contained an apartment known as the infirmary. The infirmary existed for the use of sick monks or nuns, although occasional travellers may have been admitted. Since members of the Order entered the house for life, a special place for their care in sickness and approaching death was obviously essential. The infirmary also acted as a kind of rest house where weaker brethren might recuperate after long abstinence or after the routine bleeding which their superiors regarded as an essential of healthy life. The Infirmarian was not usually a doctor but an administrator and disciplinarian. In some instances he was strictly forbidden to treat illness, although more generally charged to deal with minor ailments and sudden emergencies. 'It should rarely or never happen that he has not ginger, cinnamon, paeony and the like in his cupboard, so as to be able to render prompt assistance to the sick if stricken with sudden malady.' The drugs mentioned do not suggest a very effective armamentarium.

All orthodox medical practitioners were clerks but it does not follow that they were priests or monks. In fact, the Church authorities did not altogether approve of medical practice in the higher ranks. Some monasteries were famed for their medicine and the larger foundations often numbered a particularly skilled brother among the inmates. Smaller houses called in help from one of these or from outside the monastic system. Very occasionally a doctor was appointed at a stipend, which customarily included a robe trimmed with fur. Women doctors were not unknown and there are records of these actually attending monks and being paid a fee. Surgeons were laymen, unconnected with the Church organization. They were frequently employed and, of course, attended for regular sessions of blood-letting. Monks nursed their sick brethren, but there is mention of a class of paid attendants who may have been in the nature of male nurses.

If the part played by the monastery in caring for the laity has been overestimated, the function of the parish church and priest has been virtually overlooked. The parish church was not just a place of worship but the community centre. Only the choir or chancel was hallowed ground. The body of the church could be used for meetings and plays, just as the strong, embattled tower could be a place of refuge in troublous times. The aisles provided accommodation for unfortunates burned out of their homes and, particularly in times of pestilence, became crowded with sick people. The parish priest, although probably possessing no medical training or experience, not only visited the sick but tended them to the best of his ability. Sometimes he had to shoulder a heavy responsibility. Bishop Bronescombe charged his clergy of the Exeter diocese 'it belongs to the office of the priest to distinguish between one form of leprosy and another'.

Not only did the parish church sometimes act the part of a hospital, but hospitals resembled churches and, after the Dissolution, were sometimes employed for that purpose. The hospital known as Elsyng Spital in London became the parish church of St Alphege. Another London hospital, St Thomas Acon, ended as the Hall and chapel of the Mercers' Company. The architectural plan exactly followed that of a church. The chancel or hospital chapel stood at the east end. The nave served the purpose of a day room. Beds were in the aisles, sometimes partitioned off into cubicles. A sixteenth century woodcut of the Hôtel Dieu in Paris shows the lay-out quite clearly. A long nave, empty except for two women who seem to be comforting relatives, leads up to the altar surmounted by a large crucifix. In aisles on either side are beds each containing one or two patients. They are attended by women habited as nuns, while two more nuns sew corpses into shrouds in the foreground. A number of such hospitals still exist; good examples are to be found at Stamford and Chichester.

The organization and administration of a lay hospital was very similar to that of a monastic infirmary. The infirmarian became the warden, a kind of secretary or house governor. Physicians and surgeons were called in from outside, although some larger establishments had a paid but not full-time staff. The method of nursing varied considerably in different hospitals and at different times. It is probably true to say that the majority of 'nurses' were less ill patients. Nursing Orders do not seem to have appeared until the twelfth and thirteenth centuries, when the Crusades acted as a stimulus. In the thirteenth century the Tertiaries or Third Order of St Francis interested themselves in nursing the sick poor. These were both men and women who wore the habit of the Order but did not take vows or live in the community. The Augustinians or Austins also took charge of hospitals and Sisters of the Order worked at the Hôtel Dieu from the thirteenth century. The famous continental nursing Orders, such as the Sisters of Charity of St Vincent de Paul are of much later date (seventeenth century).

Hospitals derived from three main sources. First, every episcopal see maintained one or more houses. In pre-Norman times, the new bishop was asked at his consecration 'Wilt thou show mercy and kindness, for the

Name of the Lord, to the poor, the stranger, and all in want?' To which he replied 'I will'. The vow was translated into provision and maintenance of a building for the purpose. Second, most trade and professional guilds established houses for their aged, sick, and distressed members. Third, generous patrons founded hospitals of all kinds. By 1300, when the population of England stood at between 3.5 and 4 million, there were some 750 of these institutions, apart from the monasteries, abbeys and priories.

The foundation date of the earliest British hospital is unknown. The first authentic mention is a grant of land in 937 made by Athelstan to an already established 'Saxon hospital' at York. That 'hospitals' existed for a variety of purposes is well illustrated by another tenth-century house in Yorkshire; the declared intention of Flixton-in-Holderness was 'to preserve travellers from being devoured by the wolves and other voracious forest beasts'. In 1076 the monks of Battle Abbey in Sussex constructed outside the walls of their rising building 'the house of the pilgrims which is called the hospital'.

St Bartholomew's Hospital, London, is the first known foundation by a private patron and one of the earliest houses for the reception of sick people. According to tradition, Rahere or Rayer served as jester to Henry I; he was more probably a civil servant or royal councillor. Rayer is supposed to have found a dying family in the streets of London. Soon after this he went on a business trip to Rome and visited the now 'Christianized' Hospital of St Bartholomew on the Tiber. He vowed that he would found a similar institution on his return to London. The story may well be true, although we must remember that the twelfth century was the first of the major periods of hospital building. St Bartholomew's started work in 1123 in conjunction with a priory of Augustinians, of which Rayer became the first prior. In 1148 Bart's is described as a special resort for sick pilgrims 'languishing men grieved with various sores'.

The history of St Thomas' Hospital is open to question. In or about 1108 some kind of a hospital existed against the walls of the church of St Mary Overy, now Southwark Cathedral. This was burned to the ground a century later and reformed in 1228. First called St Mary's, the dedication was changed to St Thomas (Becket) and for a short time after its refoundation in 1552—3 was known as the King's Hospital in Southwark. The present dedication is to St Thomas the Apostle. St Katherine-by-the-Tower is unique among London hospitals because it escaped suppression. The building survived until 1827 when the whole area was cleared for the construction of St Katherine's Docks. The hospital then moved to Regent's Park. It was a royal foundation, by Queen Matilda in 1148, and this may be the reason why the Tudors did not suppress it. The largest of the London hospitals was St Mary Spital without Bishopsgate, founded by Walter Brune in 1197. It had accommodation for 180 sick poor and was valued at £400 when suppressed. The hospital with all its buildings has completely disappeared but is remembered in the district name Spitalfields.

These hospitals catered more for the needs of travellers than for near-by residents, who probably remained at home when sick or sheltered in their parish church. St Mary's, Chichester, founded in 1172 and still standing, took in both long and short stay patients:

> If anyone in infirm health and destitute of friends should seek admission for a term, until he shall recover, let him be gladly received and assigned a bed. In regard to the poor people who are received late at night and go forth early in the morning, let the warden take care that their feet are washed and, as far as possible, their necessities attended to.

A number of such hospitals came into being after the murder of Thomas à Becket in 1170. Canterbury became a place of pilgrimage. Another famous shrine, a reproduction of the Holy Family's house at Nazareth built according to plans revealed to a rich Saxon widow in a vision, stood at Walsingham in Norfolk. Pilgrims visited these shrines from all over Europe. Many were ill before starting, just as sick people make pilgrimage to Lourdes at the present day. Others fell sick on the long journey. All these needed lodgings where they could receive some kind of medical attention. Thus we find hospitals like that in the Kentish town of Strood for 'the poor, weak, infirm and impotent, as well neighbouring inhabitants as travellers from distant places'. Here pilgrims and others were cared for 'until they die or depart healed'.

Hospitals did not admit only English travellers. In 1141 Theobald, Archbishop of Canterbury, invited help for the erection of a house at Dover 'which two brethren, Osbert and Godwin, are diligently building for the reception of poor and strangers'. Several benefactors made the condition that the hospital should admit sick and needy people disembarking from cross Channel ships. By 1163 the Maison Dieu at Dover had become 'a hospitium for strangers', that is a hospital for the reception of foreigners and sick people from abroad. It served as a receiving station for sick and wounded Crusaders returning from Cyprus and the Holy Land.

The majority of hospitals catering for the sick, as we understand the term today, were lazar houses. Leprosy was the most feared of all diseases in Europe from the tenth century AD until the fifteenth. From time to time there has been considerable discussion on the exact nature of this disease, but it is now generally accepted as true leprosy. The old story of the introduction of leprosy from the Middle East by returning Crusaders cannot be entirely true, because a similar disease was known in Norway and Sweden during the ninth and tenth centuries. The time of greatest prevalence in England and France was about 1200–1350, so it can be argued that a fresh and more virulent infection appeared in Europe after the Third Crusade.

There is documentary evidence of more than 200 houses in England. They varied in size, some containing 100 or more patients, the majority between 20 and 30, many less than 5. Twelve, representing Christ and the eleven faithful apostles, was often regarded by the founder as an ideal number. Since lepers normally entered for life and since the object was segregation, a lazar house resembled a small settlement rather than a church-like hospital. A common design consisted of a group of cottages with an adjoining chapel and a cloister surrounding a green enclosure. Many were self-supporting and possessed quite large areas of fields and gardens. A lazar house generally stood on one of the main roads entering a town or village and was always sited outside the walls. Admission practically involved entry into a form of monastic life under the general rules of poverty, chastity and obedience. The master or warden was usually himself a leper. He governed through a chapter which imposed strict discipline. When lepers of both sexes were admitted, the women lived apart from the men and were governed by a prioress. In the early years, the only 'clean' members of the community were a few paid farm workers and the very important official known as the procurator or proctor who solicited alms in the outside world. Although life for the free leper must have been misery, inmates often rebelled against the restrictions imposed by their houses. In 1313 the lepers of Kingston staged a riot and actually demolished the lazar house.

Leprosy was a crime. This sounds strange to our ears until we remember that all disease was a divine visitation, usually translated into divine punishment for sin. Since leprosy produces horrible disfigurement, the sin must have been grievous. In 1318 the French King Philip V proposed to burn alive all lepers so that 'the fire might purge at once the infection of the body and of the soul'. In England the leper became outcast under the statute *De Leproso Amovendo*. The duty of deciding whether or not a person suffered from leprosy fell chiefly upon the clergy, though a jury might sometimes be empanelled to try the case. Once adjudged leprous, the sufferer lost his liberty of movement and the right to bequeath or inherit property 'The mezel cannot be heir to anyone.' (The use of the common term 'mezel' for a leper should remind us how difficult it is to make a diagnosis on mediaeval nomenclature.) False accusations of leprosy were frequently made against the testator or opposing party in cases of disputed inheritance. The Church Office contained a special form of service to be said when sending the leper forth from his home, 'The Office at the Seclusion of a Leper' as it is called in the Use of Sarum. The form was not commonly used in England but may be briefly described. The priest carried the leper from his house to the church as a dead man. There he solemnly banned the sufferer from all places of public resort, forbade him to eat or drink with the healthy or to speak to clean persons unless they stood on his windward side, nor might he ever touch a child again. The priest provided him with a bell or clapper and a dish for alms. He was given a hut, little more than a shelter of boughs, and compelled to leave his house, family and friends, to haunt the roadside, begging for food, yet warning the passer-by not to approach him closely. He existed on scraps, literally thrown at him, and, as he weakened, crept into his hovel to die.

For such an unfortunate, the lazar house must have been a place of refuge. The first known house was founded by Bishop Gundulf at Rochester in 1078. This interesting foundation escaped suppression and remains today the oldest hospital in Britain. Six years later Archbishop Lanfranc built one of the largest lazar houses at Harbledown near Canterbury for just over 100 patients. The Empress Maud, daughter of Malcolm III of Scotland and first wife of the English King Henry I, is sometimes regarded as one of the patron saints of leprosy. She founded St Giles, Holborn, for either fourteen or forty lepers in 1101, and tradition states that she took an active part in the nursing. St Giles is probably the first of the London houses.

Many more 'leprosaria' were built as leprosy increased in the thirteenth century and a number of older institutions, semi-almshouse, semi-hospital, were reserved entirely for the purpose. In 1315 the Parliament of Lincoln ordained that all houses founded for the reception of infirm and lepers be solely devoted to the latter. Admission of any other class was now often refused and bye-laws became much more stringent. In 1276 the Assize of London enacted 'no leper shall be in the city, nor come there, nor make any stay there'. The porters of the eight city gates were sworn to refuse lepers admittance and, in 1310, barbers were stationed with the porters. Barbers, acting as surgeons, claimed a special knowledge of overt disease and the authorities therefore regarded them as particularly skilled in the detection of leprosy. Berwick-on-Tweed enacted a savage law

> No leper shall come within the gates of the borough and, if one gets in by chance, the sergeant shall put him out at once. If one wilfully forces his way in, his clothes shall be taken off him and burned, and he shall be turned out naked. For we have already taken care that a proper place for lepers shall be kept up outside the town, and that alms shall be there given to them.

The incidence of leprosy probably reached its peak at the end of the thirteenth century. The will of Bishop Button (or Bitton) in 1307 shows that there were no less than thirty-nine houses in the diocese of Exeter, which then covered the counties of Devon and Cornwall. They ranged in size from a house containing eighty inmates at Pilton near the port of Barnstaple to a small establishment containing only one patient at Sancred in Cornwall. The average number of lepers in each house was thirty-four in Devon and twenty-five in Cornwall. Nine years later the City of Rochester found it necessary to provide a new lazar house, although they already possessed two. But the new hospital, St Katherine's, seems to have been for any type of long-stay patient 'if it happen that any man or woman of the City of Rochester be visited with leprosy, or other such disease that causes long impotence, with unpower of poverty, there should he or she be received'.

There was no effective treatment. Founders often sited lazar houses close to mineral springs, supposed to have particular healing powers. Harbledown, Peterborough, Newark and Nantwich are examples. Burton

Lazars, a village to the south of Melton Mowbray, is of interest. Here the house, probably built and certainly maintained by the Order of St Lazarus, stood beside a famous curative spring. St Lazarus is one of the semi-military, semi-religious Orders of the Crusades. Founded in the twelfth century at Jerusalem, its primary object was care of the sick especially lepers. It became active in France and other European countries but never took a great part in British nursing. Washing with water from a holy well or spring derived from the successful cure of Naaman as described in the fifth chapter of the second book of Kings. Diet, blood-letting, purgation, plasters and ointments were prescribed. A favourite remedy consisted of adders boiled with leeks. It is not known whether the unfortunate sufferer had to drink this revolting mixture or anoint his skin with it.

The decline of leprosy started about the year 1315 and may be connected with the widespread famine which occurred at the same time. The great mortality during the last half of the fourteenth century virtually ended leprosy in Britain. There is no new legislation after 1349. The only post-Black Death foundation is that of William Pole in 1411 on a piece of land granted by Henry IV. It is just possible that Henry himself may have suffered from leprosy, although a more favoured diagnosis is an unusually painful form of eczema caused by his gross eating habits. By the end of the fifteenth century leprosy had disappeared except in the extreme west and north of Britain. The reason for decrease is clear. In his weakened state a leper is prone to infection and unable to withstand it. Thus the Black Death caused a large destruction and the small remaining foci were wiped out by recurrent plagues. Leprosy disappeared first from the south and east, the most highly populated areas at special risk from plague, and more slowly from the less densely populated north and west. The number of lazar houses rapidly declined. That at Sherburn, Co. Durham, contained sixty-five patients. In 1434 their places had been taken by thirteen poor men unable to support themselves, but accommodation was reserved for two lepers 'if they could be found in those parts or would willingly come to remain there'. About 1360 St James' in Westminster, which used to house fourteen lepers, was empty except for a sole survivor who acted as caretaker. Henry VIII acquired this very old house, founded by citizens of London for the maintenance of 'leprous virgins', and used the stone to build part of his new palace. It is considered possible that the present St James' Chapel is the old hospital church.

The great mortality affected hospitals in two ways. First, many and not lazar houses only became redundant. Second, the weakening of church control led to abuses. The temptation to plunder the revenues of a half-empty hospital must have been great. But hospitals were still necessary as the 1414 Petition and Statute for Reformation makes clear:

> Many hospitals . . . be now for the most part decayed, and the goods and profits of the same by divers persons, spiritual and temporal, withdrawn and spent to the use of others, whereby many men and women have died in great misery, for default of aid, livelihood and succour.

All hospitals were under the patronage of somebody, the Crown, the bishop of the diocese, a merchant guild, or a private benefactor. The responsibility for use or abuse lay with the patron, although he delegated administration to an appointed warden or master. As the usefulness of a hospital diminished, so the patron became indifferent to the proper selection of a warden. Wardenship turned into a sinecure. Many wardens were non-resident and held more than one post. The Crown behaved particularly badly in this respect, often nominating men already in royal service elsewhere or appointing quite unsuitable persons who regarded the position as a stepping stone to greater preferment. There are known cases in which a boy in his early teens was given the emoluments and potential duties of warden. Patrons often purposely kept the more lucrative offices vacant so that they could enjoy the revenue.

Patrons also abused the system by demanding free accommodation and maintenance for themselves or their servants. This had often been a right laid down in the original charter of foundation. Wealthy descendants of the founder frequently used the hospital as a convenient inn when travelling with their retinue. The kings of England always exercised their right to lodge at the Maison Dieu in Dover on their journeys to and from France. The 'corrody' became another and a worse abuse because it laid a permanent burden on the income of the house. The corrody was a privilege of free board and lodging which might be granted by the community itself, or sold by an official of the foundation for his own profit, or given away by founder's kin as a reward for service. Another difficulty, becoming more complex with the passage of years, lay in the respective rights and privileges of the founder's heirs and of later benefactors. The resultant quarrel often led to an insoluble lawsuit. Many foundations came, by default of agreement, into the hands of the Crown. Crown patronage tended to limit the usefulness of a hospital because of a declaration of Edward II that royal hospitals primarily existed for the support of poor and weak persons in the King's service. Thus an increasing number developed into almshouses for royal servants.

The purpose of a hospital, with the exception of the lazar house, had never been clearly defined. It could be a geriatric unit, an orphanage, a reformatory for unmarried mothers, a rest house for travellers, an infirmary for the sick or, much more frequently, it could serve all these purposes. A certain differentiation gradually developed during the latter part of the fourteenth century. This definition of purpose formed part of a campaign against the increasing number of 'unsick stubborn knaves', the vagrants with whom Crown and municipal authorities waged grumbling warfare until well into the nineteenth century. The problem is adequately described by an ordinance of the City of London in 1359 which declared that vagrants 'do waste divers alms, which would otherwise be given to many poor folks, such as lepers, blind, halt, and persons oppressed with old age and divers other maladies'. Ten years later London ordered all 'mendicants, vagrants and pilgrims' to leave the city precincts.

The increase in vagrancy resulted in a tightening up of regulations.

The pilgrim hospitals on the roads to Canterbury and Walsingham started to refuse accommodation for more than one night except in the case of real illness. Proper inns for pilgrims took their place, many being built by the church authorities who derived an income from providing board and lodging. The Pilgrims' Inn at Glastonbury, erected by Abbot John about 1475, is a notable example. Genuine almshouses came into being largely through the benevolence of trade guilds. In 1445 the Society of Merchants at Bristol took over the premises of an old hospital and converted it into a home for aged seamen. This was, in fact, an early benefit club, members becoming eligible for admission after paying seven years' dues. Some municipalities founded similar institutions. Bubwith's House in Wells received men 'so poor that they could not live except by begging and so decrepit that they could not beg from door to door'. Distressed burgesses of Wells were to be given 'the most honourable places and beds'.

In 1379 the foundation deed of Holy Trinity Hospital, Salisbury, stated 'lying-in women are cared for until they are delivered, recovered, and churched'. The 1414 Petition and Statute describes the reception of lying-in women as a proper aim of hospital charity. Two of the greater London hospitals, St Mary without Bishopsgate and St Bartholomew's, combined obstetrics with the provision that, if the mother died, her child should be nourished at the house's expense until seven years old. About 1423 Richard Whittington endowed eight beds in St Thomas' Hospital for young unmarried women. He commanded that absolute secrecy should be observed lest the girl's chance of future marriage be embarrassed.

There seems to have been no special provision for lunatics until the middle of the fifteenth century. St Mary of Bethlehem in London, founded by Simon FitzMary in 1247, admitted patients other than the insane. In 1403 there were six male lunatics and three 'common sick' of whom one suffered from paralysis and had been bedridden for two years. But about fifty years later the hospital is described as

> A church of our Lady that is named Bedlam. And in that place are found many men that have fallen out of their wits. And full honestly they have been kept in that place and some have been restored to their health and wits again. And some have been abiding there forever, for they have fallen so much out of themselves that man cannot cure them.

Madmen are occasionally mentioned in other parts of the country. Holy Trinity, Salisbury, accepted 'the custody of the mad until their senses return' as well as lying-in women and sick persons. On the other hand regulations sometimes debarred admission of lunatics. Candidates for an endowed bed at St John's, Coventry, must be 'not mad, quarrelsome, leprous, or infected'. At least two lazar houses are known to have been converted into madhouses. One of these, St James, Chichester, gradually declined over many years until the bishop reported at the end of the seventeenth century 'it hath only one poor person, but she is a miserable idiot, in it'.

Many hospitals were closed or put to other purposes in the fifteenth century. Several, chiefly attached to Cluny in France, disappeared when Henry V suppressed the alien priories. Others were seized by monasteries. In 1479 the great Reading Abbey dissolved the hospital serving the town. The citizens complained to Edward IV that 'the house of alms was not kept', the abbot having appropriated the endowment to his own use and torn down the building. The prior and convent of Worcester suppressed St Mary's, Droitwich, took the revenues and 'expelled the poor people to their utter destruction'. Some, such as another Reading hospital, St John's, and St Bartholomew's, Bristol, became schools. Cambridge colleges received the revenue of lazar houses at Windsor and Huntingdon in 1462. Houses at Romney, Aynho and Brackley were annexed to Magdalen College, Oxford, in 1481–5.

The closure of so many hospitals caused hardship. In 1509 a scribe recorded on behalf of Henry VII 'There be few or none common Hospitals within this our Realm, and for lack of them, an infinite number of poor needy people miserably daily die, no man putting hand of help or remedy.' Henry had planned to establish very large hospitals at York and Coventry but his scheme came to nothing. However, he did convert the Savoy Palace, London, into a magnificent institution lodging 100 patients nightly. Only persons exempt from the Vagrancy Acts were received, preference being given to women in travail and men in extreme sickness.

The time had come for a drastic reorganization. As early as 1410 the Commons petitioned Henry IV to use surplus ecclesiastical wealth for various purposes, including the provision of hospitals. In 1414 the Lollard Sir John Oldcastle introduced a Bill proposing that money wasted by churchmen would be better employed in maintaining a standing army and to build 100 almshouses. In 1523 Cardinal Wolsey suggested the suppression of smaller priories and the use of their revenues for education. Shortly before 1536 the City of London drew the attention of Henry VIII to the state of their hospitals which, they said, had been provided to relieve the poor but now housed a small number of canons, priests and monks who lived solely for their own gain, paying no heed to 'the miserable people lying in the street offending every clean person passing that way'. When, in 1529, Henry suggested to the Commons that he be granted the smaller religious houses, they acceded to his demand but in regard to the hospitals expressed the hope that the king would 'reduce and bring them into a more decent and convenient order for the commodity and wealth of his realm and the surety of his subjects'. On proroguing Parliament, Henry managed to give the impression that the revenues would be applied as his Commons desired.

But, of course, he did nothing of the kind. A large number of hospitals ended with the dissolution of the smaller houses in 1536 and a few more when the greater were seized in 1539. The real year of devastation was 1545 when the Act for dissolving chantries, free chapels, hospitals and guilds swept away all the small church foundations and many lay charities. Havoc was completed in 1547 when the remainder fell to the naked rapacity of Edward VI or, rather, of his advisers. Practically every-thing went except for a few foundations belonging to corporate bodies, some houses in Crown patronage, and a few attached to a cathedral or episcopal see. Nearly all of these were almshouses. Those left did not enjoy much peace. The little St Bartholomew's Hospital in Rochester had to fight off attempts at seizure by the Crown for almost 100 years.

The monastic houses had been suppressed partly to enrich the royal treasury and partly to destroy the power of the Church. There was another reason which may have bulked large in the minds of Thomas Cromwell and Henry VIII. Vagrants were still troublesome. During the fifteenth century many hitherto powerful and active monasteries became reduced to a handful of aged monks, physically incapable of resisting the demands of 'lusty rogues' who demanded lodging and subsistence. St Cross, Winchester, was a notorious resort for bands of dangerous tramps demand-ing the dole of bread and ale supposed to alleviate the hunger of poor wayfarers. The great increase in the number of vagrants, as arable farming gave place to sheep, inevitably led to a state in which the unemployed worker (who was, after all, poor and hungry) received relief intended for the sick and aged.

Thus there was reason in the contention that monastic houses encouraged idleness. But the suppression itself released a flood of vagrants who had lived under the protection of the monasteries. In the battle to deal with this major problem, the claims of the sick, the aged, and the orphan tended to be forgotten. This is perhaps why Henry delayed so long in permitting the refoundation of hospitals. In 1538 the citizens of London made urgent petition to the king:

> For the aid and comfort of the poor sick, blind, aged and impotent persons, being not able to help themselves, nor having any place certain wherein they may be lodged, cherished and refreshed till they be cured and holpen of their diseases and sickness. For the help of the said poor people, we inform your Grace that there be near or within the City of London three hospitals or spitels, commonly called Saint Mary Spitel, Saint Bartholomew Spitel, and Saint Thomas Spitel, founded of good devotion by ancient fathers and endowed with great possessions and rents.

The Londoners asked permission to refound the hospitals themselves. If the king would grant them to the City with all their old possessions

> a great number of poor, needy, sick and indigent persons shall be refreshed, maintained, comforted, found, healed and cured of their infirmities, frankly and freely by physicians, surgeons and apothe-caries . . . so that all impotent persons not able to labour shall be relieved and all sturdy beggars not willing to labour shall be punished, so that with God's grace few or no persons shall be seen abroad to beg or ask alms.

Nothing was done for six years. During this time St Mary's lay empty, never to be reopened, and St Thomas' was deserted. Loyal sons of

Bart's, eager to show an unbroken history, have been known to state that St Bartholomew's remained open for the reception of a few lying-in women. The evidence is against them. Certainly in 1540 the hospital was 'vacant and altogether destitute of a master and all fellows or brethren'. In 1544 Henry at last replied. He now found it politic to appear as a protector of the poor and was careful to justify the suppression.

> The abuses, in long lapse of time lamentably occurring, being reformed, we have endeavoured that henceforth there be comfort to the prisoners, shelter to the poor, visitation to the sick, food to the hungry, drink to the thirsty, clothes to the naked, and sepulture to the dead, administered there. We determine to create, erect, found and establish a certain hospital.

A noble resolve indeed. But no new hospital was created, erected or founded. Only a new name took the place of an old. So there came into being 'The House of the Poor in West Smithfield of the Foundation of King Henry VIII'. All the possessions and endowments of the old St Bartholomew's had vanished into the royal maw. Now Henry returned the buildings to the City and graciously endowed them with 500 marks (about £330) a year. The citizens, not thinking this sum quite enough, raised another £1,000. With this they repaired and refitted the ancient house as a hospital of 100 beds. By the same covenant the king handed over the mad-house, St Mary of Bethlehem. It was a 'free gift' but the Mayor and Commonalty found it necessary to purchase the patronage two years later.

There had been abuses at St Thomas' just as there had been at Bart's. Most of the hospital silver mysteriously disappeared in 1536—8. The house surrendered to the king on 14 January 1540. In 1546 the citizens petitioned Henry for its reopening on a small scale, but this came to nothing and the premises remained derelict until 1551. On 12 August 1551 the City of London bought the Manor of Southwark together with the hospital and its remaining lands. The most valuable part of the endowment had been lost. In 1536 the income stood at £346 per annum. In 1551 it was only £154.17. St Thomas', although rich, had never been a large hospital; in 1538 it provided accommodation for forty patients. The citizens thought £154.17 just enough to support twenty beds and petitioned Edward VI to allow reopening on this scale. Edward replied by letters patent in 1551 'The King desiring the health of the citizens in general no less than the cure of the sick, therefore grants permission to the Mayor and Corporation to undertake the work.' It is not clear whether the City did or did not reopen the hospital in 1551.

For in the next year

> that learned and pious child, Edward VI, being, in the year of Our Lord 1552, much moved by a fruitful and godly exhortation of Master Ridley to the rich to be merciful to the poor, did suddenly and of himself send for the said Bishop as soon as his sermon was ended, willing him not to depart until that he had spoken to him.

The result of this conversation was the Royal Foundation. It consisted of three 'hospitals', St Thomas' for the sick and aged, Christ's Hospital for orphans, and Bridewell for the correction of lusty rogues. It seems to have been the original intention that all three should be housed in Bridewell, a derelict royal palace, but common sense prevailed. Christ's Hospital was provided with the suppressed Greyfriars in Newgate Street, which had already been handed over to the City by Henry and where the Franciscans had possibly managed an orphanage school for many years.* St Thomas' was repaired and enlarged to provide beds for 260 patients. The three institutions were incorporated by letters patent on 26 June 1553. The City generously provided most of the necessary money. Shortly before his death, on 6 July 1553, Edward suppressed the only remaining London hospital, the Savoy or Hospital of St John the Baptist, founded by his grandfather Henry VII, and handed over the furnishings and revenues.

It is difficult to avoid the appearance of cynicism when telling this deplorable story. The legend of the 'pious and learned child' masks the truth of a reign more rapacious than that of Henry VIII. Of the thirty 'Edward VI grammar schools' not one, with the very doubtful exception of Christ's Hospital, was an entirely new foundation. All had previously existed as charities of one kind or another. So had St Thomas' Hospital. The only certain exception is Bridewell, little better than a whipping-house for beggars and prostitutes. We cannot blame the unfortunate boy, for he was dependent upon the advice of self-seeking courtiers and certainly incapable of taking an active part in the worst piece of chicanery, the suppression of the Savoy, in the last days of his life. But we must face the facts. The whole episode of the suppression and alleged refoundation is sordid, a golden opportunity lost through sheer greed.

The Royal Foundation was not, in fact, completed until 1557. Ultra-protestant historians of the seventeenth and eighteenth centuries have inevitably cast Edward in the part of hero, Mary as villain. Mary did not undo the work of the London citizens; perhaps she feared to antagonize so powerful a body. She re-formed the Royal Foundation to

---

* V. C. Medvei and J. L. Thornton (*The Royal Hospital of Saint Bartholomew*, 1974) have stated that the Brethren of St Bartholomew's

> visited Newgate Prison, taking away small children and babies. When brought to the Hospital they were looked after by the Sisters who also took charge of foundlings and stray children. By the 15th century so many children were kept in the Hospital that a school was formed with a Latin master.

The Franciscan Greyfriars adjoined the Augustinian St Bartholomew's and was handed over to the City by Henry at the same time. There can be little doubt that the present school of Christ's Hospital derives from the Augustinian orphanage. Just as St Bartholomew's Hospital rightly claims foundation by Rahere in 1123 rather than by Henry in 1544, so Christ's Hospital should claim foundation in the twelfth century by Augustinians rather than by Edward VI in 1552.

include St Bartholomew's, St Thomas', Christ's Hospital and Bethlehem. To these she added the Savoy, which she refounded and re-endowed. The Savoy became a military hospital in 1644. Closed at the Restoration, the hospital temporarily reopened for the reception of sick and wounded seamen during the Dutch wars of 1665 and 1672. It became redundant when Charles II embarked on his design for hospitals at Greenwich and Chelsea, ending its history as a prison for deserting soldiers.

In France the Grand Bureau Général de l'Aumone des Pauvres, created by Francis I in 1544, had carried out the work which Henry VIII and Edward VI so signally failed to perform. The many ecclesiastical hospitals of France passed into the control of municipalities. Throughout the seventeenth century the French organization increasingly became a model to be copied by other countries. The Hôtel Dieu in Paris acquired the reputation of being the finest hospital in the world; even in far distant Septentrional France similar institutions on a smaller scale were founded at Quebec in 1637 and Montreal in 1644. British prosperity boomed after the Peace of Utrecht in 1713. The next years saw the rise of a wealthy middle class. They travelled extensively in Europe and were able to make comparisons. They saw not only the down-trodden peasant but also the many charitable institutions which cared for the poor in their distress.

Ideas were changing. In 1690 John Locke published his *Essay on Human Understanding*, a seminal work of the Enlightenment. Voltaire popularized the new concept in France and conceived an immense admiration for British religious toleration, freedom and prosperity. To the minds of Voltaire and his fellow philosophers, this (largely imagined) liberty of person and conscience suggested that Man is perfectible, not through Divine grace, but by his own efforts. The Perfectibility of Man, as returned to Britain, became translated into the responsibility of men for the well-being of their brothers. The new way of thinking did not affect government policy, nor was it accepted by the majority of Englishmen. The elegant Georgian facade often concealed callousness, brutality, and indifference to suffering. But, from almost the beginning of the eighteenth century, and increasingly as the century advanced, a number of private individuals became concerned for the well-being of less fortunate members of society.

Here is the origin of eighteenth century voluntary hospitals. They were founded by private individuals, rich men of the rising rentier class who, on the whole, looked for no reward in this world or the next. Their hospitals were unsupported by Church, State or ratepayers, but maintained by the benefactions of individuals and served by an unpaid medical staff. No one knows how this 'voluntary' system originated. About 1715 a group of London merchants, led by Henry Hoare the banker, drew attention to the need for a revival of 'the True Christian Spirit of Justice and Charity' among those whose duty it was to care for the poor and they called for a voluntary effort on the part of others. The group seem not to have had any clear scheme, but they opened some kind of a charitable hospital in Petty France, Westminster, in 1719. Four years later this removed to Caxton Street and started work as the first true 'voluntary hospital'. It is now the Westminster.

Hoare's group may have been influenced by the activities of Thomas Guy. Guy had been a governor of the ancient St Thomas' since 1705. In 1707 he became so distressed by the number of chronic sick who were either refused admission or discharged because nothing could be done that he rented an adjoining piece of land and erected a new block to receive them. In 1721 he decided to found and endow a new hospital on ground adjacent to the St Thomas' site. The building opened with 435 beds on 6 January 1725, just a week after Thomas Guy's death. The purpose of Guy's Hospital has been a subject of controversy ever since. Many authorities hold that he intended a hospital for the chronic sick in conjunction with St Thomas'. Chamberlayne's *Present State* for the year 1755 describes it as a 'Hospital for Incurables'. As the United Hospitals, Thomas' and Guy's worked in close conjunction until 1825, when disagreement as to the appointment of a surgeon caused a separation.

St George's at Hyde Park Corner was founded by a splinter group of Westminster governors in 1733, opening 1 January 1734. The 'London Infirmary', now the London Hospital, followed on 3 November 1740. Designed to serve the particular needs of seamen and artisans, the London has always been associated with the London docks. The last of the eighteenth century general hospitals in London is the Middlesex. No one seems really to know how it came to be founded. The date is given as 1745 when two houses in Windmill Street were rented by Mr Goodge 'to a group of Governors whom he shortly joined', their purpose being to open a hospital for the sick and lame of Soho. The governors ordered on 11 November 1746 that 'the name of the Infirmary be the Middlesex Hospital'.

The urge to found voluntary hospitals was not limited to the capital. A survey made in 1719 revealed that twenty-three English counties had no hospital accommodation at all. Eighty years later, nearly every county and many of the larger towns had its hospital or 'infirmary', founded and maintained by private benefactors. Winchester is almost certainly the earliest, although Bristol and Northampton sometimes claim priority. There are points of interest in the history of Winchester, now known as the Royal Hampshire County Hospital. Founded by Alured Clarke, a prebend of the Cathedral, it opened on 18 October 1736. Clarke encountered opposition. An Act of 1722 encouraged local authorities to establish workhouses, the cost of maintenance to be met by parish rates. Clarke's opponents argued in favour of a workhouse which, they said, would serve the purpose of a hospital and would tend to discourage malingering vagrants. Clarke made a notable reply. The Act permitted maintenance of paupers but did not provide for sick care or attendance of physicians. Therefore a hospital would serve a more useful purpose than a workhouse. If Parliament ever devised a better scheme for the care of the sick poor, then the proposed hospital would be superseded or become part of the scheme. His forecast proved correct just over 200 years later.

Alured Clarke also founded a hospital at Exeter when he was appointed Dean of the Cathedral in 1741. He had great influence upon the whole movement. For instance, the hospital at Norwich (1771) came about largely because of a sermon preached by Clarke at the opening of the Winchester Infirmary, the sermon being printed at Norwich in 1769. He regarded hospitals as more than places for care of the sick. His policy was 'to instruct the sick and reclaim the bad' during the course of their treatment. Clarke thought, and rightly, that hospitals would not only discourage the number of sick vagrants who begged from door to door, but would also reduce the number of quacks who peddled their useless remedies to the poor.

Obviously we cannot list the many general hospitals founded during the eighteenth century, but a short reference must be made to the rather strange history of Bath. Bath had been a famous curative spa for centuries. An old agreement permitted 'diseased and impotent poor' free access to the waters. The agreement expired in 1714, but 'the beggars of Bath' continued to invade the gracious Queen Anne city, sometimes terrorizing the wealthy invalids by their importunity. In 1716 Lady Elizabeth Hastings and Henry Hoare, the founder of Westminster Hospital and owner of nearby Stourhead, proposed that a hospital be erected to cope with the invasion. After some delay, a subscription list opened in 1723, Beau Nash accepting the post of collector. It proved difficult to find a suitable site and the hospital did not open until 1737. It was incorporated by Act of Parliament in 1739. Unlike other voluntary hospitals, admission did not depend upon a 'governor's letter', and the trustees accepted patients from all parts of the United Kingdom rather than reserving accommodation for the poor of Bath. However, patients from outside the city precincts had to produce a certificate of poverty from their home parish and £3 caution money to provide for the return journey or burial.

Midwifery had been practised in several mediaeval hospitals. The Middlesex set aside five beds for lying-in women in 1747 and appointed two 'men midwives' Dr Layard and Dr Sandys. Equipment was also provided 'one pound of pins, two pin cushions, two red leathers, and two child bed baskets'. Dr Sandys, with the connivance of the senior physician and chaplain, concocted a plan to transform the whole hospital into a maternity unit. They were foiled, but the committee decided to make half the bed complement available for midwifery. The first British 'hospital for women' is the famous Rotunda at Dublin, founded in 1745. Several followed in London, the earliest being the Lying-in Hospital, Brownlow Street, Long Acre. In 1914 it amalgamated with the Home for Mothers and Babies and is still active at Woolwich. The well-known Queen Charlotte's started life as the General Lying-in Hospital in 1752. A number were founded in provincial towns, the earliest probably being Princess Mary Maternity Hospital, Newcastle-on-Tyne. All these eighteenth-century foundations were for 'married women'.

Paediatrics had an unfortunate history in the eighteenth century. Dr George Armstrong founded a Dispensary for the Infant Poor in 1769. His dispensary was very successful but failed to attract subscribers and had to close in 1783. Armstrong had hoped to develop his dispensary into a hospital for sick children and it is perhaps fortunate that he failed. The Foundling Hospital of London was established by Captain Thomas Coram and started work in 1741. All eighteenth century hospitals were founded with good intentions but it cannot be said that standards of sick care and administration reached a high level. The Foundling Hospital, in its first years, was little better than a place for the disposal of unwanted children. Of 14,934 children received below the age of two months, no less than 10,389 died. A foundling hospital established in Dublin had an almost incredible record. During the period 1775—96, 10,272 infants were admitted. Of these, only forty-five survived. A leading medical historian, Dr Fielding H. Garrison, remarked that the eighteenth century hospitals 'sank to the lowest level known in the history of medicine'. This is, perhaps, an overstatement but it was to be many years before the hospital developed from a house for lodging the sick into an institution for the cure of disease.

3 Medical education: The birth of a profession

The practice of medicine has from time immemorial been shared by orthodox and unorthodox attendants. Until very recently the larger part of the population depended upon unorthodox, that is unqualified practitioners. An unorthodox practitioner is not necessarily a charlatan. The bonesetter, for instance, had an intimate knowledge of skeletal anatomy and based his practice upon that knowledge. He became a charlatan only when he strayed outside his 'speciality', for example if he pretended to cure a gastric ulcer by manipulating his patient's spine. The difference lay—and lies—in education. The modern orthopaedic surgeon performs many of the manipulations of the bonesetter, but his training is not confined to skeletal anatomy and orthopaedic surgery. His medical education covers so wide a field that he is, or should be, competent to deal with ailments which lie outside his limited speciality. We can therefore define the orthodox practitioner as a person who has received a regular and broad education or training in all aspects of medicine.

But the orthodox practitioner will always regard the unorthodox as something of a charlatan even if he confines his practice to a limited sphere. Medical education implies the specialized training of persons destined to be members of a closed group. Anyone who practises outside this group will be regarded with suspicion. There are many things to be learned from unorthodox practice, but these real and useful skills will then be regarded as part of orthodox training. Having been absorbed, such knowledge will be confined within the group and not disseminated. Since there are advantages in belonging to a closed group, any arts or skills, whether acquired from outside or developed within, will be jealously guarded.

The group was originally familial, gathered knowledge being passed from father to son. The apprentice took the place of the son, his master that of the father. The 'descendant' of Aesculapius became the 'follower' of Aesculapius, organized guilds or societies of physicians known as Asclepiads. The most famous of these guilds existed on the Island of Cos about 420 BC. Often accorded the title of the 'Coan School', this Asclepiad was not only a closed group of physicians but a very efficient teaching unit, possessing an excellent library and training the apprentices to observe, to record data, and to make careful diagnosis before instituting treatment. Further, the guild of Cos evolved an ethical code. It is probable that in all known forms, there are clauses inherited from older guilds and others which are later additions. This is the Hippocratic Oath, taking its name from Hippocrates, the most famous physician of the Coan school or, perhaps, from the name by which the guild was known. There are many versions, differing only in detail. Here is a typical example:

> I swear by Apollo the healer, by Aesculapius, by Hygeia, by Panacea and by all gods and goddesses, making them my witness, that I will fulfil this oath and indenture to the best of my ability and judgement.
>
> I will hold my teacher in this art equal to my own parents; I will share my livelihood with him; I will provide his necessities if he is in want; I will look upon his offspring as my own brothers and I will teach them this art, if they wish to learn, without any fee. I will teach by example, oral instruction, and by all other means to my sons, the sons of my teacher and to pupils who have sworn the Oath of a Physician but to no one else. I will treat the sick to the utmost of my ability and judgement but never to their hurt or for any wrong purpose. I will never administer a poison if asked to do so nor will I suggest any such thing and I will not assist a woman to procure an abortion, but will keep both my life and my art pure and holy. I will not use the knife, not even upon sufferers from the stone, but will give place to those who practise this craft. Into whatever houses I enter, I will enter to help the sick and will abstain from all intentional wrongdoing and harm and especially I will not seduce any man or woman, bond or free. And whatever I see or hear when attending the sick, or even apart therefrom, which ought not to be told, I will never divulge but hold as secret.
>
> If I hold to this oath and do not break it, let it be mine to enjoy life and art alike with good repute among all men at all times. But if I break this oath and fall into wrongdoing, may the opposite be my fate.

The Hippocratic Oath has provided the basis of approved professional conduct for 2,000 years. Seduction of a patient and malpraxis, or the treatment of a patient to his hurt, are still professional crimes for which a doctor can and probably will be struck off the register. As late as 1966 medical correspondents in the public press seriously invoked the promise to keep secret any information while attending the sick when a senior physician published a book divulging the medical history of his famous patient, Sir Winston Churchill. But if we examine the Oath critically, we see that the essence is a promise to support members of the group, to confine teaching of the art to a closed circle, and not to reveal the mysteries to anyone outside that circle. It embodies a high ethical standard and closely resembles the oath taken by a Freemason. The masonic oath promises to observe a code of behaviour but the essence is never to divulge the secrets except to a brother. Thus the Hippocratic Oath ensured a 'closed shop' and this closed shop persists today in the differentiation between the privileged registered practitioner and the unregistered quack.

The Oath did not apply to all members of the medical profession as we understand the term today. Many authorities maintain that the clause 'I will not use the knife . . .' is a late interpolation but, even so, it has been part of the Oath for 1,000 or more years. This dichotomy within the profession arose early and persisted until comparatively recently. The surgeon did not find a place in the physicians' guild. The physician has always tended to regard himself as an intellectual and the surgeon as an artisan. A physician trained in the schools, a surgeon by apprenticeship. Until late in the eighteenth century, the story of medical education is the story of the physician. Unless this is appreciated, it is not possible to understand the difference between physician, surgeon and apothecary, the internecine struggles, and the emergence of a unified profession.

The schools of Alexandria (331 BC) and of Cairo were large and trained students in the art of medicine on a more extensive scale than did the guilds. They influenced development more in the Near East than in Western Europe. The first European school, to which we can properly give the name, developed in the small seaside town of Salerno, about fifty-six kilometres south of Naples. A company of physicians a 'civitas Hippo-cratica' settled here in the ninth century AD. The place was already a well-known health resort, easy of access, lying close to the Greek-speaking lands of Sicily and Southern Italy where some knowledge of Greek medicine lingered on. It is thus understandable that physicians should have settled in Salerno, but it is more difficult to explain why so great a school should have developed. State warred against state; medicine lay under the dominion of Christian Church and Arabian scientist. Yet the Salernitan school was both international and interdenominational. The legend of foundation by four masters, Elinus the Jew, Pontus the Greek, Adale the Arab and Salernus the Latin Christian, cannot be accepted as historical fact but serves to underline the truth that the school opened its doors to all irrespective of language, nationality or creed.

Little is known of the teaching but it must have been more catholic than later schools. Salerno produced not only good physicians but skilful surgeons such as Roger of Palermo and Roland of Parma. A very interesting point is that women graduates are known. They were probably mid-wives rather than physicians or surgeons. Of the four named 'ladies of Salerno' (Trotula, Abella, Rebecca, Constanza) Abella wrote two books while Trotula has provided a mystery. She may not have been a person but a book, from the title of which all Salernitan midwives derived the appellation 'Trotula'. She has entered nursery lore as 'Dame Trot and her cat'.

The great age of Salerno was in the eleventh and twelfth centuries. In 1140 King Roger II of Sicily issued an edict forbidding the practice of medicine without proper examination by the Salernitan faculty. In 1224 his grandson, Emperor Frederick II, laid down regulations which may be looked upon as the first medical curriculum. The intending student must be over twenty-one years of age, of legitimate birth, having already studied logic for three years. The medical course lasted five years, with an additional year of practice under the supervision of a senior man. After examination, the successful Salerno graduate took an oath based upon that of Hippocrates but containing an additional promise not to keep an apothecary's shop. This clause later became generally adopted in the form of prohibiting the physician to dispense his own medicines. The graduate then received a ring, a laurel wreath, a book and the kiss of peace. He was accorded the title of either 'doctor' or 'magister'. It is commonly believed that the title 'doctor' for a medical man who may not even hold a university degree derives from Salerno.

Salernitan teachers produced an extensive medical literature, about 100 books in all. These were probably the text books used in the school and continued to influence medical education long after the importance of Salerno as a teaching centre had waned. The best known is a kind of popular guide to health, written in double rhymed hexameters. Titled *Flos Medicinae* or *Regimen Salernitanum*, the work became widely disseminated through translation into many languages. It passed through a number of editions and was expanded from an original of less than 360 verses to ten times that number. The author and date of writing is uncertain, probably not before 1130. Salerno started upon its long decline early in the thirteenth century when Frederick II instituted a university at nearby Naples. The famous school gradually decayed until no better than a purveyor of bogus degrees and was closed by order of Napoleon on 29 November 1811. No trace now remains.

Medical education passed to the multi-faculty universities, of which Bologna and Padua in Italy and Montpellier in France became well known for the excellence of their teaching of medicine. Oxford and Cambridge offered courses from a quite early date. In 1284 we find Archbishop Peckham ordering that study of medicine should cease at Merton College, Oxford, on the ground that it was contrary to the founder's statutes. At about the same time a number of physicians settled in Cat Street by whose efforts a regular faculty of medicine became established in 1311—12. The regulations were similar to those of Salerno and probably reached Oxford from Bologna. The long courses of study demanded a preliminary seven years reading Arts, but this included philosophy. Lectures and disputations on the theory and practice of medicine occupied the next four years. The candidate then presented himself for examination by Masters, who issued a licence to practise in Oxford, and only in Oxford, for two years. During this probationary period, the doctor must still attend lectures but was permitted to gain clinical experience by attaching himself to an established physician, a provision similar to that of Salerno and not unlike the pre-registration post of today. Thus the Oxford student of medicine could only obtain his degree after thirteen years training. The regulations for the Cambridge doctorate resembled those of Oxford, but there seems to have been no regular teaching in medicine until late in the fourteenth century.

Only a minority of medical practitioners, and by no means all physicians, underwent this arduous course. Since all 'orthodox practitioners' were clerks and came under episcopal jurisdiction, the bishops exercised control over orthodox practice. The third grade in the minor orders was that of exorcist, who had the power to cast out unclean spirits. Only a bishop could authorize elevation from one grade to the next. It therefore follows that a bishop could confer upon any man who had served in the second grade of acolyte the powers of exorcist. Such is the genesis of 'the bishop's licence', the authority of the bishop to practise medicine. The high mortality among clerks during the plague-ridden second half of the fourteenth century resulted in a proliferation of quack doctors who seized the opportunity to make money from all classes of society. The regular practitioners took fright. In 1421 came the first attempt to control medical practice by licence. Either the universities or the graduate physicians petitioned Henry V to enact that only those possessing a degree should be licensed and that others should be required to undergo examination before continuing any form of practice. The proposal came to nothing but may have suggested action to Dr Gilbert Kymer, Chancellor of Oxford, in 1423. Kymer nearly changed the history of the medical profession when he established a conjoint faculty of medicine and surgery. His project met with no success and ended within a few years.

English medicine had fallen into a low state by the beginning of the sixteenth century. A few physicians possessed a degree from an Italian, French or English university. A tiny minority of surgeons had been licensed after examination by one of the universities to practise in any part of England. Church domination had degenerated to such an extent that clerks who practised under licence from a bishop were often illiterate. The bulk of the profession—trade is a better term—consisted of barber-surgeons who belonged to a number of guilds, only permitted by guild-law to practise locally. On the fringe there hovered a multitude of quacks and a number of semi-quacks, such as the wise women who filled the part of midwives and paediatricians, and the grocer-apothecaries, sometimes called pepperers, who compounded and dispensed drugs and who often advised treatment.

There can be no doubt that this anarchy resulted from the general break down of ecclesiastical prestige. Just as care of the sick passed out of the Church's hands to be reformed, albeit on a very limited scale, by the Crown, so the Crown undertook to infuse some order into the confusion of medical practice. Henry VIII had many faults but, perhaps because he was a notable amateur physician, proved a good friend to doctors. In 1511–12 he instigated the first Medical Act, which starts with the preamble

> Physic and Surgery is daily within this Realm exercised by a great multitude of ignorant persons as common artificers, smiths, weavers and women who boldly and customably take upon them great cures and things of great difficulty in the which they partly use sorcery and witchcraft to the grievous hurt, damage, and destruction of many of the King's liege people.

The Act made it an offence to practise physic or surgery unless the practitioner was a graduate of a university or had been licensed by the bishop of his diocese after examination by a panel of experts. Unlicensed practitioners were made liable to a fine of £5 per month. The Act served to establish a fairly respectable body of medical men, although it did nothing to enforce proper training.

Graduate physicians and guilds of barber-surgeons lay outside the scope of the Act. Thomas Linacre, an Oxford graduate and MD of Padua, had served as tutor and physician to Prince Arthur, elder son of Henry VII, and continued to act as one of the physicians to Henry VIII. In 1518 Linacre petitioned Henry and obtained from him a charter establishing a Company of Physicians which became the Royal College of Physicians of London in 1551. The charter empowered the Company to examine and license physicians throughout the kingdom, to control practice within seven miles of London, and to ensure the purity of drugs sold by apothecaries. The surgeons soon followed the physicians. Thomas Vicary, a barber-surgeon of Maidstone, moved to London and rapidly rose to fame, becoming a surgeon to Henry VIII in 1535. Five years later, in 1540, he secured the king's assent to a union of all the scattered guilds in England. The United Company of Barber-Surgeons could impose fines upon unlicensed surgeons only in London. Of greater consequence is the small detachment which the charter effected between surgeon and encumbering barber. Separation did not become complete until 200 years later, but in 1540 the surgeon was no longer required to act the part of barber, while the barbers were ordered to restrict their surgical operations to dentistry. The charter also entitled the Company to receive the bodies of four executed criminals each year for the purpose of dissection and study of anatomy.

These measures served to organize the trades of physician and surgeon. Unfortunately it soon became apparent that there were not enough to meet the demand. In 1542 Parliament enacted the so-called 'Quacks' Charter'. This term is a misnomer, because the Act simply recognized a situation which could not as yet be amended. The 1542 Act exempted from the penalty prescribed in 1512

> divers honest persons, as well men as women, whom God hath endowed with the knowledge of the nature, kind, and operation of certain herbs, roots, and waters, and the using and ministering of them to such as be pained with customable disease.

Exemption could only be claimed by those who charged no fees except for providing the herb itself. During the reign of Charles I this provision was upheld in a famous judgment when the College of Physicians brought an action against a herbalist named Butler.

While the legislation of Henry VIII brought some sort of order into chaos, it widened the rift between physician and surgeon. The former remained a university graduate. Although the College of Physicians issued licences to non-graduates, it did so grudgingly and would only accept graduates as Fellows. Further, members of the College made the strange claim that they had a right to practise surgery as part of physic, and their claim was upheld in 1540. At first glance, this might seem to promote unity and such may have been the intention of the 1540 enactment. But in fact it had an opposite effect. Since the physician had no intention of practising surgery himself, he translated the decision into a ruling that the surgeon was a subordinate who performed his operations under the physician's direction. The surgeon deeply resented this attitude and became increasingly antagonistic to the physician. About 1580 an enlightened surgeon named John Banester tried to heal the breach and to unite surgery with medicine which, he maintained, must benefit both. 'Some of late' wrote Banester 'have fondly affirmed that the chirurgeon hath not to deal in physic. Small courtesy it is to break faithful friendship, for the one cannot work without the other, nor the other practise without the aid of both.' Sensible words, but Banester failed to move either his surgical brethren or the entrenched physicians.

A third party now engaged in the struggle. Just as surgeons were encumbered by barbers, so the apothecary suffered from a long standing association with grocers. Apothecaries sold fine groceries as well as drugs; grocers included in their stock items more properly described as drugs. Oriental spices were used as medicines but also to flavour foods and as preservatives for winter meats. A 'cordial' is a strongly alcoholic liquor, distilled with herbs, and sweetened. To the apothecary, a cordial was a cardiac stimulant, as the word implies. To the grocer, it meant a heartening drink, a liquer rather than a medicine. Thus there came a large measure of overlap and the apothecaries took exception to the more powerful grocers stealing their trade. When the College of Physicians, acting under the terms of their charter, appointed four Censors to inspect the drugs and merchandise of the apothecaries and to destroy anything harmful, their anger was increased.

No one knows who initiated the move to separate apothecaries from grocers. Credit is often given to King James I and this may be well deserved for James, besides being a walking pathological museum, interested himself in the compounding of medicines. In 1606 they were incorporated as an adjunct or separate section of the very large Grocers' Company and, eleven years later, became an entirely separate Society under a charter granted by the king. The little Society of Apothecaries, a City Company, encountered opposition from all sides. The Grocers tried to reabsorb them, and were frustrated by the personal intervention of King James. The Lord Mayor of London cold-shouldered them for seven years. The physicians obstructed their advance in every possible way. The apothecaries won their battle because they, rather than physician or surgeon, served the public as general practitioners.

Even today a person suffering from a minor ailment will not trouble his doctor but call on the chemist to suggest 'something for my cold'. The law permitted an apothecary to dispense drugs; the College of Physicians strongly protested when he started not only to dispense but to prescribe. Since it is undesirable to prescribe a drug without knowing the nature of the disease, apothecaries were forced to 'advise', that is to enquire into the patient's symptoms and attempt a diagnosis and prognosis. The apothecaries argued that they were entitled to do so by virtue of the 1542 Act, provided they charged only for medicine and not for advice. Many apothecaries charged exorbitant prices for their medicines and thus circumvented the Act without damaging their own interests. But it was common to charge the poorer classes only for the cost of their medicine and so the apothecary became the poor man's doctor. In 1687 the physicians tried to arrest this development by binding all Fellows and Licentiates to treat the poor free of charge. In 1696 they started to found dispensaries at which the poor received not only advice but cheap medicine, an attempt to undercut the apothecaries. These moves proved unsuccessful and in 1703 the physicians decided to obtain a judicial decision by prosecuting an apothecary named Rose. The physicians won in the lower court but a decision of the House of Lords found for Rose. The right of an apothecary to act as a doctor had been established.

Surgeon and apothecary trained by apprenticeship alone and their training was severely practical. The lordly physician could, and often did, receive his degree without examining a patient. His training was entirely academic and almost entirely classical. It could be little else because the universities were academic and classical in their teaching. In 1575 William of Orange founded a university at Leyden as a reward for the city's magnificent defence against the Spaniards in the previous year. The University of Leyden opened its doors to all students irrespective of nationality or creed. In this it differed from Oxford and Cambridge, which would admit only members of the Anglican Church, and the majority of European universities, under the control of Roman Catholics. All teaching was in Latin, the common tongue of educated men. Leyden became an international university, attracting Catholics from Protestant countries, Protestants from Catholic, and the many British who did not belong to the established Church. Students came from England, Scotland, and the American colonies, drawn by the excellence of Leyden's teaching of anatomy.

The history of the Edinburgh medical school is closely bound with that of Leyden. In 1660–1 Robert Sibbald spent eighteen months at Leyden and returned to Scotland where he founded the College of Physicians of Edinburgh and became the first professor of medicine in the Town's College, as the university was then called. Two more Leyden students, James Halket and Archibald Pitcairne, joined him as teachers of medicine, both later following him in the chair. In 1692 Pitcairne accepted a professorship of medicine at Leyden. He stayed for only one year but had as a pupil Hermann Boerhaave. Having served as a very successful junior lecturer, Boerhaave was appointed professor of botany and medicine to the University of Leyden in 1709.

Little or no clinical experience could be gained in the English universities and the same was true of Leyden until Boerhaave became professor. He had been allotted care of twelve beds in the town hospital. Now he used these for teaching purposes to such good effect that students flocked to his clinics—the first time that the word can be rightly employed to describe medical teaching in a European university. Boerhaave introduced bedside medicine into the training of a physician.

John Monro, a surgeon, had been another of Pitcairne's students at Leyden. Monro conceived the idea of establishing a medical school in conjunction with the Town's College or University of Edinburgh on the same international lines as that of Leyden. To this end, he trained his son, Alexander Monro, as a surgeon and anatomist, sending him to study under Boerhaave and under the famous William Cheselden at St Thomas' Hospital in London. John Monro remained in Edinburgh working on his son's behalf. In 1719, when his son was only twenty-two years old, John Monro secured his appointment as professor of anatomy. Alexander Monro taught anatomy and surgery with great success for thirty-eight years, and was followed in the chair by his son and grandson. In 1725, when Monro primus was obviously on the road to fame, four leading Fellows of the College of Physicians of Edinburgh petitioned the Town Council for appointments as professors. All four were successful. In the following year Joseph Gibson received a chair of midwifery, the first in any university.

The College of Physicians had for some time been urging the foundation of a hospital. By 1729 sufficient money had been raised to make a start. On 25 August 1736 George II granted a charter incorporating the hospital as the Edinburgh Royal Infirmary. Right from the beginning the Infirmary worked in close association with the University. Eight of the twenty managers were, by statute, to be physicians and surgeons, of whom at least three must be professors. It is clear that the founders' primary intention had been to provide a clinical teaching school; in this respect the Edinburgh Royal Infirmary differed from any other eighteenth century hospital foundation. With a well-qualified teaching staff and a wealth of clinical material, Edinburgh became the mecca of the aspiring student. Scottish qualifications were not recognized as licences to practise in England; the attraction of Edinburgh lay in systematic teaching and clinical instruction. Classes were immense; in 1828 the famous (or notorious) anatomist Robert Knox regularly lectured to a class of over 500 students. He had to repeat each lecture three times as the theatre held a maximum of 200. Knox's assistants often spent sixteen hours on end in the dissecting room.

The eighteenth century foundation of hospitals in London and the larger English provincial towns resulted in a number of small teaching centres. The rules of the Royal College of Physicians obliged Fellows to attend the poor without charging fees. The physician found it easier to honour his obligation by accepting an unpaid hospital appointment. He soon realized that the clinical material available in the wards attracted apprentices. Hospital managers discovered that ambitious young men would, for the same reason, pay quite large fees to attend the sick as 'house pupils'. A modern medical student unconsciously recalls the past when he says that he is 'on Dr Blank's firm'. The firm consisted of the physician, his small band of apprentices, and the house pupil who acted the part of a present-day house officer.

Systematic teaching in the English hospitals was impossible because the Company of Barber-Surgeons insisted on their prerogative of dissecting human bodies, and would allow no dissections outside their own Hall. They could not prevent anatomical demonstrations at the Royal College of Physicians, but the number given was quite insufficient and attendance strictly limited. In 1745 William Cheselden, one of the most enlightened of eighteenth century surgeons, secured the separation of the barbers. Cheselden and a few of his colleagues visualized the new Surgeons' Hall as a teaching centre for London. His health failed before the project came to anything, but his idea was pursued by William Hunter. In 1746 Hunter started anatomical classes at a house in Covent Garden, where he was later joined by his more famous brother John. The Hunter school became popular and twice moved to larger premises.

William Hunter now embarked on a more ambitious scheme. In 1763 he petitioned Lord Bute, First Lord of the Treasury, for a lease of Crown land on which to build at his own cost a school of anatomy, museum and library

> or, if His Majesty's known love of the polite arts, and his benevolence towards mankind, should suggest to him a design of establishing an academy on a more extensive plan, Dr Hunter would be still more happy if what he now proposes for the advancement of one science, might be made a small part of an institution worthy of the British nation and a British King.

Hunter, in effect, suggested the foundation of a medical university in London. The Government proved sympathetic and explored the possibilities of various Crown properties, Scotland Yard, the Savoy, St James' Park, the Royal Mews. But they procrastinated. Hunter, who had promised £6,000 towards the project, wrote withdrawing his offer unless a site was agreed within three months. George III, who seems to have been genuinely interested, was not amused by this pistol held at his head and the Government refused to pursue the matter.

Even now, Hunter might have succeeded for Lord Shelbourne suggested a public appeal and offered £1,000 as a starter. Hunter, resentful and disappointed, would not consider the offer and decided to proceed alone. He bought 16 Great Windmill Street, had it rebuilt to his own plans, and started a course of lectures in 1767. Hunter was joined by a number of teachers but the school remained a private enterprise. Lecturers bought a share and recouped themselves from their pupils' fees. Many famous medical men of the early nineteenth century started their successful careers in Windmill Street: Matthew Baillie, Sir Charles Bell, Professor Brande of the Royal Institution, Peter Mark Roget of the *Thesaurus*, are some. Beginning as an anatomy school, it rapidly expanded to provide formal courses in chemistry, surgery and medicine. This, the first medical teaching school in London, virtually ceased to exist in 1833, although sometimes claimed as the ancestor of the present Middlesex Hospital Medical School.

The success of Windmill Street encouraged formation of a number of private schools which may be classed as good, bad and indifferent, the majority falling into the last two categories. By the end of the eighteenth century it became apparent that English medical education varied considerably in standard and that the average was disturbingly low. Oxford and Cambridge awarded both degrees and licences, but training approached the farcical. Sir Isaac Pennington of Cambridge, described as 'a stately physician of the older school' held the post of Linacre lecturer in medicine for fifty years, professor of chemistry for twenty, and the Regius professorship of medicine for twenty-three years. During the whole of this multiple tenure he gave not a single lecture in any subject. Oxford awoke from torpor during the latter part of the century, an anatomy school being opened in 1767 with a small, active medical school centred on the Radcliffe Infirmary, but relapsed into ancient inertia after a few years. Possession of a university doctorate had become nothing but a status symbol and a necessary qualification for the Fellowship of the Royal College of Physicians. Any graduate with ambition almost invariably took an additional course at Edinburgh and often attended a London hospital as well.

A rapidly increasing population demanded more doctors and there were too few available. Towards the end of the century practitioners in country towns started to form societies, partly to discuss scientific subjects and partly to protect their own interests. Some of these made surveys to find out the kind of medical attention provided in their districts. One such enquiry in the North of England showed that, of 266 practitioners, only 68 had received any form of medical education. Another in Lincolnshire revealed a total of five physicians, all trained at Edinburgh, eleven surgeons and apothecaries trained by apprenticeship, twenty-five druggists, of whom only one had served an apprenticeship but who all acted as doctors, sixty-three midwives, not one of whom had been trained, and forty quacks without any education at all. Patterns similar to this were commonly found in country districts and the rising industrial towns.

Social change also demanded more doctors with a higher standard of education. The Industrial Revolution greatly increased both numbers and wealth of the middle class. The physician attended land owners and aristocrats. He entered the house by the front door. If the services of an apothecary or a country surgeon were required, he used the tradesmen's entrance. Only the physician and a few distinguished surgeons could claim the title of 'gentlemen'; the large remainder were tradesmen. Wealthy manufacturers declined to entrust the bodies of themselves and their families to the ministrations of uneducated practitioners and demanded something better. Their demand accounts, in part, for the great influx of Edinburgh graduates but the number was not sufficient to meet the need.

Internal jealousies aggravated the position. The three trades of physician, surgeon and apothecary were separate but their several duties were undefined. Each arrogated to itself the right of practising all branches of medicine. Each accused the others of trespassing upon its own preserve. In the middle years of the eighteenth century a number of licentiates tried to enforce a more democratic constitution upon the Royal College of Physicians in an attempt to win for themselves the right to practise in any part of the country instead of being confined to London and seven miles around. In 1789 a severe epidemic of typhus at Manchester induced the managers of the Infirmary to increase the medical staff by the appointment of more apothecaries and surgeons. This move angered the physicians. One of their number, an unusually liberal-minded man named Thomas Percival, wrote a short pamphlet in which he outlined a code of behaviour which should be observed by the various branches of medical practitioner who formed a hospital staff. His booklet was published under the title *Medical Ethics* for private circulation in 1794 and generally in 1803. Percival's subject was not 'medical ethics' as we understand the term today, but *medical etiquette*. The fact that Percival was asked to publish his small book nine years after its initial private circulation reveals the anxiety of the more reasonable doctors to find some method of working in amity with their potential rivals.

To men like Percival, to the ambitious licentiates, were opposed the arrogant physicians determined upon retaining their ancient privileges. These were the bearers of 'the gold-headed cane', the Fellows, who held all the lucrative appointments, who attended the Court circle and the aristocracy. Their real knowledge of medicine was often inferior to that of the humble apothecary who treated the sick poor and possessed no qualification other than apprenticeship. The physicians prided themselves upon their classical learning, spoke and wrote in a form of dog Latin which had degenerated into abracadabra and served to hide ignorance. Percival trained at Edinburgh, where he came under the influence of William Cullen, the first physician to teach in English. Percival's friend Thomas Beddoes, a brilliant but eccentric physician of Bristol, urged that medical writings should be not only in English but in terminology understandable by the layman. Himself an MD of Oxford, who had held a lectureship in the University, Beddoes attacked his fellow physicians 'of the cane, the peruke and the other distinguishing insignia of the profession'. He poured scorn upon their pretensions. Speaking through the mouth of one of these anachronisms, Beddoes put the case in a nutshell

> Seeing into what confusion things have run, why should we be surprised if the *licentiate* comport himself as if he were on a par with the *fellow*? Why wonder that we who have been matured in the regular discipline of episcopalian universities, should be held in scarce higher estimation than those who have but just had time to lick up a mouthful of the husks of science at some presbyterian seminary in the North?

The move for reform therefore came from three main groups; the new rich who demanded better attention; a group of younger physicians, particularly those trained at Edinburgh, who saw the danger of a divided profession; the mass of licentiates, surgeons and apothecaries, who not only demanded recognition but also were alarmed by the increase in the number of unqualified practitioners. In the early years of the nineteenth century Sir Joseph Banks, President of the Royal Society and lately a manager of the Apothecaries' Physic Garden at Chelsea, instigated an enquiry into the best method of reforming medical education. It is probable that the Apothecaries took the lead because of Banks' close connection with the Society. In 1815 they secured an Act declaring that all apothecaries in England and Wales, except those already in practice, must be examined and licensed by the Society after serving a five years' apprenticeship. The Society was empowered to prosecute offenders.

The Apothecaries Act of 1815 marks the dividing line between the old and the modern systems of licensing. The ancient corporations could only exercise control in London and the environs but the new powers given to the Society permitted control throughout the Kingdom. It seems that nobody, except for one member of Parliament, understood that the Act gave the whole control of medicine into the hands of the Apothecaries. For they had power to prosecute *anyone* who practised without their licence. Fortunately they behaved with wisdom. But they seized the opportunity offered and imposed regulations to be observed by candidates before examination and licensing. The Apothecaries demanded not only a five years' apprenticeship but also certificates showing that the apprentice had attended two courses of lectures in anatomy and physiology, and two courses in the theory and practice of medicine. The major innovation was the rule that a candidate for examination must have 'walked the wards' of a recognized hospital for at least six months.

In 1800 the old Company of Surgeons became the Royal College of Surgeons. The Napoleonic Wars greatly increased the number required by the armed forces. Since warfare is one of the greatest schools of surgery, the majority had better practical training than ever before. When peace came, they were not content to accept the ill-defined and minor place which they had previously held in the medical hierarchy. They demanded at least equality with the apothecaries, yet the Society now controlled practice. The College therefore tried to obtain for themselves similar privileges by Act of Parliament, but the attempt failed. Their only course was to come to private agreement with the Society, and to raise the status of their diploma by following the Apothecaries' regulations. The requirements of the two bodies could be met by an additional course of lectures in surgery and an additional six months spent in the wards of a hospital. Although many pupils still confined themselves to the MRCS or the LSA, it became customary for any ambitious young man to seek qualification from 'college and hall', that is Membership of the Royal College of Surgeons and the Licence of the Society of Apothecaries. So developed the 'physician and surgeon' or fully qualified general practitioner.

While there is no doubt that the Act of 1815 greatly enhanced the prestige of the practitioner and that the Apothecaries made wise use of their powers, the educational system which emerged was by no means satisfactory. Regulations demanded certificates but did not insist upon supervision or a set curriculum. Evasion became common. Lecturers often accepted their fee and issued a certificate at the beginning of the course, thereafter caring little whether the pupil attended or not. Pupils combined their courses of lectures with 'walking the wards'. This was in some ways a better system than our present one, for the intelligent student could correlate anatomy and physiology with bedside teaching. But the method was a bad one for the majority, because, lacking efficient direction, they tried to compress too many subjects into too short a time.

The Act caused a proliferation of private schools which were nothing but cramming establishments for the Apothecaries' exam. These schools offered the regulation courses, often conducted by excellent teachers, but they exercised no supervision over their pupils. The primitive medical schools, developing in conjunction with the larger hospitals, suffered from the same fault. Lack of supervision produced 'the medical student', exemplified by Mr Bob Sawyer and Mr Benjamin Allen in Dickens' *Pickwick Papers*. It must be remembered that the student had already served an apprenticeship. Many of these young men resented the six months of walking the wards before examination and licensing. Many others simply looked upon the time as a holiday between the toil of apprenticeship and the arduous life of a practitioner. A lad was often bound when only twelve years old. Youths in their late teens, reared in sleepy country towns, found themselves flung for six months or a year into a great city among a crowd of their own type, without any organized recreation and, all too often, without advice. Little wonder that they became notorious as the wildest set in town, drunken, lecherous, making night hideous with their pandemonium. The bad name acquired by hospitals during the first half of the nineteenth century can be largely attributed to the reputation of their medical students.

The hospitals possessed neither facilities nor disciplinary apparatus to cope with the horde of young provincials which descended upon their wards after the Act. Consultant physicians and surgeons still retained their select band of indentured apprentices and house pupils, who paid large fees for their privileges. Obviously these received the best teaching. Since they acted directly under the direction of their masters, they and they only gained practical experience from performing minor operations and taking an active part in diagnosis and treatment. The large remainder, the ward-walkers, could only learn by looking on. Many hospitals confined their tuition to attendance at ward rounds and asking questions. A few hospitals did not even permit the latter.

For all its faults the 1815 Act, as interpreted by the Society of Apothecaries, proved remarkably successful. The extent of its success can be measured by the number of men who submitted to the Society's regulations and acquired the licence. In the years 1842—4 only sixteen licences were granted by the universities and thirty-seven by the Royal College of Physicians. The remaining English licences, 953 in number, were granted by 'college and hall', that is by the Royal College of Surgeons and the Society of Apothecaries. The Act produced a new class of educated general practitioner. Because the Act suffered from imperfections, it was these new young men who themselves demanded revision. The demand expressed itself in an agitation for a more orderly method of training and in the Medical Reform movement.

Benjamin Golding founded the Charing Cross Hospital in 1821 with the expressed purpose of providing a university education for medical students. Charing Cross can therefore claim to be the earliest of the true London 'teaching hospitals', initiated with the primary purpose of training doctors and with the secondary purpose of caring for the sick. But Charing Cross never became a university in its own right. Seven years later, in October 1828, a large group of men including Thomas Campbell, Jeremy Bentham, Henry Brougham and Joseph Hume founded the 'University of London' or University College. The 'godless college of Gower Street' aroused the wrath of the Establishment who replied with King's College, Strand, in 1831. Both colleges had small medical departments from the beginning. University College acquired an associated hospital for teaching its students in 1834 and King's College founded its own hospital in 1840.

Thus, in 1840, a few London medical students were undergraduates, studying in multi-faculty colleges. No real university system existed and the old lack of supervision remained. Teaching was geared to the requirements of the Society of Apothecaries. It is of significance that the medical professors took the lead in demanding a degree-conferring University of London. They were not content to act as mere tutors for the limited curriculum required by the Apothecaries' regulations. They saw the danger inherent in a system which apprenticed a young lad for a term of five years, condemned him to a short period of restricted instruction, and loosed him upon the world as a 'professional gentleman' without a general education. The professors strove for a wider basis of education and they succeeded in their struggle. The University of London, incorporated by charter of 1836, offered degrees in medicine two years later, although these were not accepted as licences to practice until 1854.

The Anatomy Act of 1832 added some much needed dignity to medical teaching. Before 1832 a student had little opportunity of dissecting the human body himself, and demonstrations were surrounded with an aura of suspicion. Schools acquired few bodies by legitimate means, the great majority being furnished by 'resurrection men' who rifled graves and purveyed corpses to the teachers. The watchman's hut and stout iron railings still to be found in some churchyards are a reminder of the days when a knowledge of anatomy could only be gained by means of this ghastly trade. The Burke and Hare scandal in Edinburgh which broke the anatomist Robert Knox, and the less notorious murder of the boy Carlo Ferrari, followed by the attempted sale of his body by John Bishop to Professor Partridge of King's College in November 1831, induced Parliament to legislate. The Anatomy Act empowered the Secretary of State for the Home Department to issue licences permitting the lawful acquisition of bodies for purposes of dissection. The Act not only made teaching much easier but put an end to the evil reputation of anatomy schools.

The medical student was also in process of being tamed. In 1842 Professor Robert Bentley Todd addressed a powerful open letter to the Council of King's College in which he proposed a collegiate system for the medical department, similar to that which obtained at an Oxford or Cambridge college. His full scheme could not be implemented for lack of funds, but he succeeded in instituting the offices of Dean and Medical Tutor, the former to maintain discipline and the latter to advise. In 1843 the more wealthy St Bartholomew's Hospital opened the first hostel for students. Other medical schools followed both examples, particularly after the University of London offered degrees. Although the licence of the Apothecaries remained the most popular qualification for many years, and their regulations therefore had to be obeyed, apprenticeship gradually assumed a place secondary to medical school training. The change was rendered inevitable by the great nineteenth century advances in scientific knowledge, which could no longer be taught by an untrained master to his apprentice in the surgery or at the bedside.

The Medical Reform movement existed in embryo during the last years of the eighteenth century but was given a powerful stimulus by the new generation of respectable, educated practitioners. They found their champions in Thomas Wakley and Charles Hastings. Wakley founded the *Lancet* in 1823. From the start this radical journal served as the rallying point for those who attacked the lethargy of the old medical corporations and who demanded reform. Wakley, a militant agitator, himself led the onslaught. The number of small, local medical societies which had been a feature of the 1790s rapidly increased during the early years of the nineteenth century. Most originated as lending libraries, circulating books and journals of medical interest, but soon developed into clubs for scientific discussion and social intercourse. From here was but a step to mutual protection. After 1815 many of these societies extended their aims beyond the protection of members to a general campaign for advancement in the social status of doctors.

In 1816 Charles Hastings founded, or possibly resurrected, the Worcester Medical and Surgical Society. His Society was largely responsible for the agitation which preceded the Anatomy Act of 1832. It is entirely due to the outstanding drive and personality of Hastings that a provincial medical society, far removed from the centre, should have exerted so great an influence. In 1828 he started publication of *The Midland Medical and Surgical Reporter*, and four years later broadened the basis of the old Worcester Society to become the Provincial Medical and Surgical Association. The Association, which embraced physicians, surgeons and general practitioners, held its first annual convention at Worcester in 1832. Hastings, an indefatigable worker in the cause of medical reform, received a knighthood in 1850. In 1855 the Society which he founded changed its name to the British Medical Association.

The above short paragraph purposely omits any account of the struggles between rival societies. All pressed for reform but they differed in the means to be used and the type of reform required. The College of Surgeons came under particularly fierce attack, led by the pugnacious Thomas Wakley. In 1843 the College surrendered and prayed a new charter. It became the Royal College of Surgeons of England, responsible for the control of surgical practice throughout the Kingdom. The old self-perpetuating governing body disappeared to be replaced with a Council, democratically elected by a new body of Fellows, 300 in the first instance. These were selected from the leading surgeons of the day, but Fellowship by examination soon followed. We can with certainty date the modern highly qualified surgical specialist from the first examination in December 1844 when twenty-four candidates passed.

This triumph did not satisfy the reforming party. The Poor Law Amendment Act of 1834 dealt a severe blow to the status of practitioners in country and industrial areas. The Act required Boards of Guardians to appoint parish or union doctors. In wealthy districts the practitioner could ignore the Guardians and still make a living. In country villages and the poorer industrial towns, his only hope of existence was by acting as parish doctor. Tight-fisted Boards of Guardians drove the hardest possible bargain. In many areas they cared little whether the 'doctor' was qualified or not; the man who would accept the lowest wage, sometimes as little as £20 a year, received the appointment. The Apothecaries had the power to prosecute anyone who practised without their licence, but detection was difficult and prosecution expensive.

Agitation for reform therefore came chiefly from the new class of educated general practitioners. Not only did they fear a proliferation of unlicensed quacks but they resented the pretensions of the older generation. They might only be licentiates of the Society of Apothecaries, but were better trained and more competent to practise than their alleged superiors, the graduates of ancient universities. They knew this and they demanded equal privileges. For this reason the majority favoured a single licensing authority and one medical qualification which would entitle the holder to practise any branch of medicine in any part of the country. As a corollary, any person who did not hold this qualification would be debarred from practice and liable to prosecution.

The reformers did not win their battle, but cholera did some of the work for them. The great epidemics of the mid-nineteenth century forced government action, simply because it became necessary to appoint Medical Officers of Health, and there existed no register of qualified practitioners from which these officers could be selected and their qualifications checked. This is the genesis of the 1858 Medical Act. The declared purpose of the Act was to enable the public to distinguish between qualified and unqualified practitioners. It placed all the existing licensing corporations under the control of a new and powerful body, the General Council of Medical Education and Registration, now known as the General Medical Council. Their first duty was to compile a Register of qualified practitioners. The next and more important duty was to ensure that qualification could only be attained after suitable courses of study and clinical training. The Council, formed by appointees of the Crown, from the corporations and from the universities, was subject only to the Privy Council which could intervene or reverse decisions if the occasion demanded.

The Act satisfied no one, least of all the Reformers. It failed in two major respects. First, the Reformers had demanded that unqualified persons be debarred from practice. The Act allowed for the prosecution of such persons *only* if they posed as qualified practitioners. Hindsight shows us that there were two good reasons for mitigation. In the first place it is an infringement of liberty to debar a patient from seeking the aid of a herbalist, a spiritual healer, or other unorthodox practitioner if he so desires. In the second place much para-medical treatment and advice was still given in 1858 by the village parson or lady of the manor; it would be difficult if not impossible to determine where friendly help ended and 'doctoring' began. Secondly, the Act did not impose the single qualification and single licensing body which the majority of Reformers desired. The negotiating committee made an attempt but encountered so much opposition from the medical corporations that they abandoned the scheme. There are many who believe that an opportunity was lost, for the continuing existence of some twenty licensing bodies perpetuated the academic snobbery which the Reformers had rightly sought to end. Had the Act imposed a single qualification, as is the case in the United States, the struggle of the new 'ancillary specialities' to attain equality with the old-established physician and surgeon during the twentieth century would have been less arduous.

But the Act worked. For the first time in history a whole calling submitted itself to a single governing body possessing almost judicial power. Since the General Medical Council assumed the right to discipline, it was enabled to formulate an ethical code to which all registered practitioners must conform. This ethical code is a high one and it has raised the social prestige of the doctor in public estimation. We can now observe the paradox that the 1858 Medical Act, intended to protect the public rather than the doctors, has in its implementation transformed the medical trade into the medical profession and benefited the doctors as much as the public.

4 The years of plague

Any history of medicine must primarily be the story of a battle waged against illness. It is also the story of disease itself and, from the point of view of social consequences, this aspect may be of equal importance. A number of diseases have affected the welfare or actually retarded the development of civilized man. They have appeared seemingly from nowhere, caused vast pandemics or exerted a prolonged insidious destruction, and have faded out either for reasons unknown, or through social changes, or by defeat at the hands of scientists and medical men. So far as we know, illnesses of one kind or another have always been with us; no sooner does one type disappear or suffer defeat than another takes its place. The cancers which, despite intensive research, cause so many deaths today, held only a minor place in the disease pattern of the fourteenth century.

Cancer arouses fear and the fear is sometimes more agonizing and more difficult to treat than the cancer itself. Leprosy was the most feared of all diseases during the three centuries after the Norman conquest. A terribly disfigured leper, in the last stages of his insidious illness, should arouse only pity. But it is natural for the ordinary person to recoil in horror and to fear contamination. The terror of leprosy pervaded society and accounts for the seemingly heartless legislation against people whom we now know to have been innocent and unfortunate victims of a chance infection. But what were the chances of becoming infected? The numbers of lepers cannot have been large and it is almost certainly true to say that the incidence never reached more than 4 or 5 per 1,000 of the population. Such an incidence is minute when compared with the mortality caused by later epidemics. We are justified in assuming that the fear rather than the prevalence of leprosy induced harsh treatment.

The low incidence of leprosy and the disproportionate fear aroused suggests that the 250 years following the Norman conquest must have been more healthy than the next three centuries. There is good evidence that this is true. Sickness associated with famine appears to have been the only type of major epidemic. This is probably typhus fever which tends to be prevalent in dirty communities suffering from gross malnutrition. Reports suggest local rather than nationwide epidemics. In the thirteenth century, a period of intense arable farming, we can identify with certainty only one famine on a national scale, that of 1257—9. In the years 1066—1300 population growth appears to have been steady and fairly rapid. There are no reliable figures and such estimates as have been made cannot be regarded as accurate. The Domesday survey suggests a figure of not more than 1.25 million in 1086. Calculations based on increased acreage under cultivation and the size of communities have supposed a population of between 3.5 and 5 million in 1300, a mean of 4.2 million being commonly accepted. By 1380 the number calculated on the Poll Tax returns of 1377 had fallen to under 2.5 million.

It is necessary here to emphasize a self-evident truth. Immigration and emigration barely existed. In mediaeval Britain, population could only rise if the number of live births exceeded the number of deaths. Population could only fall when the number of deaths exceeded the number of live births. It follows that, during the period 1086—1300 more people were born and survived to bear children than the number who died. This is not the case for the years 1300—80. The normal process of birth continued and so did the normal process of death. But at some time during the period there must have been an abnormal mortality. This could have been caused by deaths greatly outnumbering live births throughout the eight decades or by a short period of vast mortality which caused a temporary halt in the increase of population, thus producing the loss of almost 2 million suggested by the estimates for 1300 and 1380. The loss undoubtedly occurred and, despite the arguments of some modern writers notably the late Professor Shrewsbury, there is little reason to doubt that an abnormal mortality did occur in the years 1348—50.

If so rapid and so large a loss of manpower occurred in so short a time, it is reasonable to suppose that the catastrophe effected some social change. We know that social upheavals did occur at the end of the fourteenth century. But it is unwise to assume that these resulted solely from the mortality of 1348—50. Change began almost a century earlier. From 1200 onwards an increasing acreage came under plough. A glut of labour and a shortage of land developed in the cultivated area around existing settlements; arable gradually extended on to marginal ground which today would be regarded as unsuitable for corn. At that time England was a corn-exporting country. Then, about the year 1300, something happened and no one really knows what that something was. Possibly a long period of continental weather, hot summers and cold winters, gave place to the wetter and less extreme Atlantic system. Perhaps continual arable farming on marginal land, without adequate manuring or proper rotation, so exhausted the soil as to make corn growing uneconomic. Sheep, which assumed the first place in agricultural economy during the fifteenth and sixteenth centuries, had already become a quite important branch at the end of the thirteenth, at a time when shortage of manpower had not yet dictated a type of farming requiring only a small labour force. Whatever the underlying reason may be, recession had begun in the early years of the fourteenth century, followed by a fall in the standard of living and of population growth.

The system of land-tenure imposed by Feudal Law already showed signs of strain in 1348. Money played little part in an economy which, theoretically at least, depended upon service. Increase of coin during a time of agricultural prosperity enabled a number of more ambitious villeins to extend their acreage, free themselves from service dues, and employ labour at a wage. During the boom years of the thirteenth century there was quite considerable buying and selling of land by free peasants and exchange or leasing by the unfree. A potential danger lay in the anomaly that poorer peasants of the less highly cultivated areas had a better chance of freedom, while the more wealthy peasants of predominantly arable lands not infrequently found their bondage increased.

Even after the lapse of 250 years, the ruling class still remained foreigners. Differences of speech daily betrayed them. The peasants used dialects derived from their Germanic and Nordic forefathers; the noble and churchman spoke in Romance languages, French or Latin. Not until 1362 was English made the language of the law-courts and in 1363 Parliament was opened in English for the first time. The City of London issued its first English proclamation in 1384 and the earliest known will written in English dates from 1387. Translations by John of Trevisa, the *Piers Plowman* of William Langland, the *Confessio Amantis* of John Gower, and the first worthy English poetry by Geoffrey Chaucer, are all productions of the late fourteenth century. By 1348 the long French War had embittered the peasant against all things French. To him, war implied high taxation, enforced service, and the son who failed to return. It was not the great game of chivalry played by the upper class, to whom the opposing knight was less an enemy than a courteous rival. The detested and oppressive forest laws brought lord and peasant into continual collision. In 1348 a man might be mercifully hanged for murdering his wife but could still be flayed alive for killing one of the king's stags.

The Church formed part of both the temporal authority and the land-owning class. People and Church were already falling out of sympathy before 1348. There are many reasons: the administrative power exercised in the State by abbots and bishops, the greed of an institution owning nearly one-third of the country's total acreage, the scandalous sale of pardons and indulgences, the grinding poverty of a hard-worked parish priest compared to the fatted leisure of abbey and cathedral, these are some. The Church cried out for reform, as some English churchmen admitted, but reform was not possible because the British offshoot was only one small part of a continental organization possessing immense authority. To the minds of many Englishmen, if not in fact, both Church and State were foreign systems imposed upon native institutions by a minority. Discontent lay close to the surface in the England of 1348, although not openly expressed by an uncommunicative people. It is for this reason that the Black Death acted as a very strong catalyst, speeding up and intensifying changes which had already begun.

'Black Death' is a comparatively modern expression. The late Professor Shrewsbury, who preferred the older 'great mortality' held that

Mrs Markham, the children's historian, coined the term about 1820. If this be so, Mrs Markham used 'black' in its secondary sense of 'atrocious', for she wrote of 'a most terrible pestilence; so terrible as to be called the black death'. There seems no point in discarding a term which has been in common use for over a century, although it may have no long sanction and is not descriptive. Here, the 'Black Death' will denote the pandemic of 1346—50 and later outbreaks will be referred to as 'plague'.

The Black Death was bubonic plague, a virulent infection of rodents, transmitted by fleas which are parasitic on both rats and men. The causative organism is *Pasteurella pestis* and the most lethal vector is the Old English or Black rat because this animal is companionable with man and there is more chance of fleas transmitting infection from one host to the other. But the bubonic type does not itself cause vast pandemics. In certain unknown circumstances, the infection will assume a pneumonic form, a virulent pneumonia which does not require the bite of a flea to infect the human, but can be transmitted directly from one person to another by droplet infection. Both forms will coexist in pandemics, but it is the pneumonic type which produces a very rapid spread, a high incidence and, since the pneumonia is usually fatal, a large mortality.

Bubonic plague is not normally endemic in Northern Europe. So far as is known, European countries had only once before been attacked, in the years 540—90 during the reign of the Emperor Justinian of Byzantium. The Plague of Justinian caused a very large mortality, recurred over a period of half a century or more, and then retreated to its ancient fastness in Manchuria and lay dormant for 800 years, although there may have been small, infrequent epidemics on the Mediterranean seaboard and in the Near East. But plague was not the only new disease to be encountered after 1348. The next two centuries are remarkable for the introduction, or perhaps reintroduction in a more lethal form, of several diseases previously unknown or of a mild type in Europe. Syphilis is one and the sweating sickness is another. *Variola major*, the dangerous form of smallpox, may be a third. The reason is not far to seek. Until the fifteenth century contact with the East could only be by the age-old caravan route, a journey taking at least a year. There was no contact at all with lands across the Atlantic. In 1453 when the Ottoman Turks sacked Constantinople and drew an iron curtain across the land route, Western Europe sought a road to the East by way of the African coasts and across the Atlantic Ocean. The voyages pioneered by Prince Henry the Navigator and Christopher Columbus brought back new or refreshed diseases in addition to more welcome amenities.

Without knowledge of the cause of disease, without proper quarantine regulations, without effective pest control, European ships proved a constant source of infection until the beginning of the twentieth century. Syphilis, introduced to Europe from Africa or the West Indies about 1490, was at first highly infectious and covered the whole continent in a swiftly spreading pandemic, then lost its initial virulence, only to be refreshed when carried by ship to unprotected communities. Yellow fever, the dreaded yellow jack, travelled from Africa to America or vice versa and appeared in English ports. The innocuous measles almost wiped out the inhabitants of Polynesia when introduced to the South Pacific. Recurrent plagues of London during the sixteenth and seventeenth centuries caused high mortalities because shipping brought fresh, lethal strains of *Pasteurella pestis*. We can observe a similar mechanism today. Influenza, now an endemic disease in Britain, is constantly being refreshed by imports which flare into nationwide epidemics.

We must seek an exotic source for the Black Death and we find it at the trading station of Caffa (now Theodosia) on the Russian shore of the Black Sea. A Tartar horde brought the infection with them from some focus in the East, invested the town, and transmitted the plague to a small band of Genoese traders who had taken shelter. In the winter of 1346—7 the garrison evacuated Caffa by sea, carrying the plague to Genoa. From this European focus, the Black Death spread rapidly through Italy, France, Britain and Germany to North Russia where it joined a second wave, originating from Tartar bases on the Black and Caspian Seas.

The Black Death first arrived in England at the small port of Melcombe, now part of Weymouth, on the coast of Dorset. It was carried by ship, probably from a Gascony port, and appeared in the middle of June 1348. The plague seems to have been static and local for a time, which suggests a rat—flea—man cycle, but the pneumonic form must have developed within two months. This form then swept rapidly through the counties of Dorset and Somerset, westward to Devon, northward to Bristol, where it first appeared on 15 August, on to Gloucester and then eastward to Oxford and London, infecting the capital at the beginning of November. There now came a short respite during the winter months when rats, fleas and fourteenth century humans all tended to be less active. The Black Death broke out with redoubled vigour in the spring. Oxford, infected before November, did not experience its highest mortality until May. London suffered only a few deaths during winter, but the number increased rapidly in March, rose to a peak in April and May, and then gradually declined.

The Black Death had now come to the edge of the Eastern Counties and Midlands, the wealthiest and most thickly populated area of England. Spread became very rapid, reaching Norfolk in March and York during the latter part of May. By the end of May, the whole of the south, east and midland districts had been attacked and the rate of progress slowed in the more thinly populated north and west. Ireland received infection by ship in 1349, but Scotland and Wales escaped until 1350. In the west of Cornwall, in north-west England, in mountainous districts of Wales and Scotland, where villages were few and roads almost non-existent, quite large areas remained unaffected.

But the Black Death did not inflict a uniform mortality even in severely affected areas. We can see what must have happened in some villages by considering the well documented 'Plague of Eyam' in 1665—6. Eyam in Derbyshire had about 350 inhabitants and received plague through a box of old clothes sent from London in September 1665. The disease must have remained in the rat—flea—man cycle until June, for only 29 people died in the nine months. In June it changed to the pneumonic form, 19 people dying in the last three weeks. The villagers now proposed to flee but were dissuaded by the vicar, William Mompesson. As the result of his well-meaning but absurd advice, 57 people died in July, 78 in August, 24 in September and 15 before 11 October when the plague ceased. In all, 259 villagers died, leaving 33 alive.* Only one man is certainly known to have fallen sick and escaped with his life, but there must have been some others.

The Eyam figures, if applied to the whole of England in 1348—50 would suggest that between 80 and 90 per cent of the population perished, a not impossible mortality in a community struck by the pneumonic type of plague. The wide divergence of monastic death-rates suggests a quite different pattern. There were places like Christchurch, Canterbury, in which only four deaths occurred among eighty monks, probably from causes other than plague. The great abbey of Crowland is another which seems to have entirely escaped. At the other end of the scale are foundations such as Luffield, which lost all its monks and novices, St Mary Magdalen at Sandon where all perished, and a nunnery at Wolthorpe with only one surviving sister. Between these two extremes come places like St Albans, which lost forty-nine out of sixty monks, West Malling where twenty-one out of twenty-nine died, and the abbey of Meaux in which one-fifth of the inhabitants survived. It is a fair assumption that village mortality patterns resembled the monastic.

The pattern accords with the known behaviour of pneumonic plague, one of the most infectious and lethal of diseases. Very few members of an infected community will escape and, of those attacked, the majority will die. When a village became infected, the death rate was high, but equally in both underpopulated and densely populated areas there must have been a number of villages which escaped, as the monastic records suggest. Thus, some villages retained their pre-1348 population intact, some were entirely, although often temporarily, wiped out, and there were some where less than a quarter of the inhabitants died. It is quite impossible to make even an approximate estimate of the number who perished during the Black Death. But the actual number is of little significance, provided it was sufficiently large to exert a major effect upon the available labour force. The reason for the events which followed the

---

* Mathematically-minded readers will notice that Mompesson's figures do not tally. It is known that a number of villagers fled, which accounts for the discrepancy between a population of 'about 350' and a total of 259 dead plus 33 survivors equalling 292. There are 22 deaths unaccounted; these may represent the mortality among those who fled and were buried outside the village, or perhaps Mompesson could not keep an accurate record during the terrible months July and August.

Black Death is to be found, not in the number who died, but in the pattern of death.

The pandemic was followed by a short period of unwonted plenty. Money, corn, cattle, were all more freely available than in 1347. This is the time of which Langland writes, when peasants who had been content with stale vegetables and cold bacon would eat nothing except fresh meat and fish, served hot unless they catch a chill on the stomach. The excess occurred because the fields had been sown, the cattle had not suffered from disease, and fewer people remained to be fed. Thus food became plentiful and cheap in the producing areas. Since manpower was in short supply, manufactured goods and materials which must be transported over long distances rose steeply in price. For instance, that essential commodity salt, by which alone meats could be preserved for winter use, rose from 3½d. a bushel in 1347 to 1s. 2d. in 1350. The landlord depended upon agricultural products for his income and prices had fallen. He used more manufactured and imported goods than the peasant, and he now had to pay more for them. Initially the landlord suffered while his workers' standard of living improved.

Had the Black Death inflicted a uniform pattern of death throughout the country, the difficulty would have resolved itself within a short time. A smaller population would have tilled and fed off a smaller area. There would have been a sufficient labour force for manufacture and cartage. In the years before 1347 there had been a glut of labour and a shortage of land; a uniform mortality would have rectified the discrepancy. In 1350 there still existed a labour glut and a land shortage in those manors not seriously affected by the Black Death. The position was only reversed on those manors which had experienced a high mortality. It is this wide difference which accounts for agrarian trouble. The landlord of a badly affected group of villages possessed perhaps a quarter of the labour essential to cultivate his lands. Only a few miles away there might be a manor which still owned more labourers than it needed. The situation was complicated by the many villeins who had already commuted their services for a payment in cash or kind. They, too, required farmworkers, though on a lesser scale than the landlord. If such a villein lived in a badly affected area he would be unable to hire workers and so be unable to make payment. His landlord, being himself desperate to find labour, then required him to resume service.

During the Black Death, the English peasant became more mobile, initially the purposeless movement of a frightened people seeking escape from disaster. An element of purpose appeared after 1350. Reason dictated a certain removal of excess labour from an unaffected area to an affected one. Action on this line seems to have been confined, or almost confined, to the Church, the largest landlord in the country, owning manors in all areas. The majority of landlords found it more convenient to tempt labour by offering a wage. The labourer soon found that he could *ask* a wage and that he would receive it if he went to a manor short of workers. In 1349—50 the purposeful movement of villeins who had hitherto been tied to the manor whose lord they served became more rapid.

Such movement undermined the system of feudal tenure, which could not survive unless the peasant, whether bond or free, consented to work his lord's demesne in return for leave to cultivate strips of land. Overall scarcity of labour and the rise in wages forced up the price of both manufactured goods and agricultural products. The central government took swift action. The 1349 Ordinance and the Statute of Labourers in 1351 aimed at preventing all kinds of worker from transferring their services from one employer to another, the primary target being the peasant. But the Statute also sought to peg prices at the 1347 level, and here the law affected employer equally with employed. The Statute not only forbade the worker to demand higher wages but the employer to offer them. The landlord in a badly affected area found himself in an impossible situation. Some broke up their demesnes, leasing the ground in small plots for a money rent. The majority strove to enforce their feudal rights by demanding the full service due, which implied service by villeins who had already commuted. This was no breach of law, commutation being a privilege and not an entitlement. It had arisen because, in the glut of labour before 1348, some lords had found it more economical to let land and pay for labour instead of depending upon the rather unwilling service due to them. Now the situation had radically changed.

The laws made necessary by this changed situation gave rise to hardship and a great deal of resentment. But the Statute of Labourers did succeed in restoring stability. The national economy started to recover. It even became possible in 1355 to recommence hostilities with France, halted by the truce of 2 May 1349. Wages and prices never fell to the 1347 level but at least ceased to rise. The labour shortage continued because, since all age groups had been affected in 1348—50, the normal death rate cancelled out the number of children reaching working age. Population rose slowly as the number of live births outstripped the number of deaths. A statesman surveying the national scene in 1360 might have thought the worst to be over.

There are no records of serious epidemics between 1350 and 1361. That of 1361 is the most controversial in the history of epidemiology. There is no need to enter the controversy here. For the purposes of this paragraph, we shall assume that the 1361 epidemic was a recurrence of bubonic plague and that one attack of plague will confer at least a limited immunity against a second. Both assumptions would be challenged by many epidemiologists and medical historians. The one certainty is that the disease, whatever its nature, caused a particularly high mortality among children, becoming known as the *pestis puerorum*. In 1361 there still remained a number of people who had not been infected by the Black Death, and in addition, there was the whole age group of one to eleven, born since 1350 and so possessing no immunity at all. The latter suffered heavily and is the essential group because, if we take the age of starting effective work as fourteen, they would have provided recruits for the ten-year period 1365—75. In the fourteenth century average expectation of life stood at not more than forty years. It follows that the same decade also saw the death of many labourers who had started work before 1348, that is who had been born before 1334 and had experienced the custom of service existing before the Black Death.

The land—labour crisis worsened throughout these years, partly because of the great loss of children in 1361 and partly because recurrent epidemics prevented recovery. The Statutes could no longer hold down prices and became a weapon directed solely against the labourer. The peasant not only found his bondage increased to the detriment of his own farming but saw vast tracts of land uncultivated. He fought back against his lord with the strike, refusing the unpaid labour he owed to his master. The landless class simply left a manor where the landlord declined to offer higher wages. Landlords, desperate for labour, hired these vagabonds without asking awkward questions. Their former masters strove to drag them back by legal process. Since judges, lawyers, and juries all belonged to the landowning class, the scales were weighted against the labourer who asked higher wages rather than the master who offered them.

Increasing discontent culminated in the revolt of 1381. This was triggered by the unpopular Poll Tax of 1377 but the insurgents' demands reveal a more or less concerted programme of agrarian reform. They sought to exact the commutation of all servile dues in return for a 'fair rent' of 4d. an acre. The 1381 rising was almost confined to East Anglia and the Home Counties, the heavily populated agricultural areas where the Black Death and subsequent plagues had caused the highest mortality. After an initial success, the rebellion failed largely because the leaders trusted an inept king and his terrified counsellors, and was followed by bloody reprisals. Neither Peasants' Revolt nor the brutal reaction could solve the underlying problem. As trouble spread from the Home Counties into the North and West, relatively unaffected by the great mortality, landlords began dimly to understand that the old system had become unworkable. From 1381 onwards came an increasing tendency to break up the demesne. The lord retained ownership of the land but ceased to farm it himself. Gradually there emerged the new pattern of landowner and tenant-farmer, depending for his labour upon a landless proletariat.

Just a century after the Black Death, in 1455, the feudal nobles took advantage of a dynastic struggle to conduct a great land-grabbing operation and, in so doing, committed mass suicide. After the Wars of the Roses the ex-villein, now tenant-farmer, emerged as the landlord and the wool baron, the first because he had become wealthy enough to buy up the estates of his ruined lord, the second because shortage of labour forced him to turn over his increased acreage to sheep. So prevalent and so profitable did sheep-farming become that shortage of labour again reverted to glut in the early years of the sixteenth century. 'Your sheep, that were wont to be so meek and tame and so small eaters', wrote Sir Thomas More, 'now, as I hear say, be become so great devourers, and so wild, that they eat up and swallow down the very men themselves.'

These 'new men' came to power under the Tudors. Unlike their predecessors they were of the same villein and Saxon stock as the class which they employed and later governed. Although often arrogant and bitterly resented, this new aristocracy never formed a closed caste, as did their counterparts in Europe. Since younger sons were forced to make a living by engaging in trade or in a profession, the squirearchy found it easy to receive recruits from these classes into their own. Such a continual fusion made for social stability and prevented the kind of class warfare by which, and by which alone, the power of a closed aristocracy could be overcome.

The Revolt did not have agrarian reform as its sole object. A large section of the insurgents demanded seizure of Church lands or total disendowment. The mob, during its temporary occupation of the Tower of London, captured Simon Sudbury, Archbishop of Canterbury, and struck off his head amid the plaudits of a large crowd. Such an act would have been unthinkable a century before, when the threat of eternal damnation still operated as an effective deterrent. The murder is symptomatic. The Church had lost both power and prestige during the years 1348–81. As a landowner on a vast scale, she suffered material damage and, in trying to restore the damage, became as unpopular as any landlord. Reduction of manpower harmed the organization and, since the best of the clergy stayed with their stricken flocks, death struck hardest at the conscientious and self-sacrificing. The career priest fled. Langland records that 'sithen the pestilence time' London has been filled with country clergy touting for high places instead of ministering to their parishioners.

Loss of prestige harmed the Church to a greater extent. An institution which reserves to itself all medical learning, all power to cure or to intercede, must justify those claims at a time of exceptional mortality or lose credibility. The utter failure of the Church to avert mass suffering during the Black Death and subsequent plagues destroyed confidence in its miraculous powers. The surprising fact is not that the confidence of the ordinary man was shaken but that the Church survived relatively unharmed. Dissatisfaction took the two usual forms of revolt and counter-revolt. There is visual evidence of the latter in the extensive, largely unnecessary, church-building and rebuilding during the late fourteenth and fifteenth centuries. Revolt, expressed as dissent from the established organization and practices of the Church, became widespread. Dissent assumed so bizarre a pattern in Europe that Norman Cohn suggests the world may have narrowly escaped a Second Coming, a revelation vouchsafed to some unknown leader of the Flagellants.

The Flagellants were not a Black Death phenomenon. They had already appeared in Italy and Germany during the severe famine-sickness of 1258–9 and small bands roamed about the continent thereafter. But it is only in the years 1347–9 that we can truly speak of 'the flagellant movement'. They attracted a large following and formed an organized society which lived under discipline, wore a habit, and conducted their strange rite according to set rules. The Flagellants were, of course, masochists but, in the main, not of the kind who derive sexual satisfaction from suffering. Most belonged to the type who undertake the sort of work which the ordinary man will regard as dangerous, sickening and unrewarding. Since plague was a manifestation of God's wrath, the Flagellant sought not to punish himself but to divert divine anger from his fellows. The rumour of pestilence, rather than pestilence itself, instigated his anxiety to offer himself as a scapegoat. Gradually the purpose changed. From intercession the Flagellants turned to revolution, dedicating themselves to purification of their world by stamping out the enemies of Christ and by reforming Church and State. Their violence and their numbers constituted a very real threat which demanded stern action by the established authority. Pope Clement VI who had at first welcomed the movement as a desirable mass penance, issued a Bull condemning flagellation in October 1349. The sect was cruelly persecuted and finally driven underground.

The Flagellants never gained a strong following among the more phlegmatic English. Here dissent took a less flamboyant though ultimately more dangerous form. It had its origin in two natural types of reaction to mass disaster. The years after the Black Death resembled the years between the two World Wars, characterized by a general relaxation of moral values and a cynical, unhappy pursuit of pleasure; this is the natural reaction of a people whose faith has been shaken. Always, in these recurrent times of doubt, there will be a core of serious minds who believe that salvation lies, not in refusing God, but in approaching more closely to Him. Such men demand the essence of religion and discard the worldly trappings.

This was the teaching of John Wyclif and his followers, the Lollards. Wyclif dared to question the hitherto unchallenged power of Holy Church. But he desired closer communion with God. He advocated a vernacular Bible and Order of Service, which could be readily understood by ordinary people, not solely by priests and the educated class. He attacked the sale of pardons and indulgences, the worship of relics, and endowment of masses for the dead. He went much further, for he attacked the hierarchy itself. Wyclif denied that the authority of the Pope stemmed from St Peter and so from Christ. He held that the Papacy derived its immense power from the Caesars, that its sovereignty was temporal and not spiritual. Up to this point, Wyclif commanded a large body of support drawn, not only from common people, but from the nobility, the friars, and from many lesser clergy who disapproved of wealthy prelates. Then two things happened. First, in 1379 Wyclif attacked the doctrine of transubstantiation. Second came the Peasants' Revolt of 1381 which hardened the ruling-class mind against any form of unorthodoxy. Increasing reaction changed tolerance to active persecution. The Lollards were never entirely defeated but persisted throughout the fifteenth century as scattered groups, almost but not quite confined to lower-class inhabitants of towns. Just as John Huss of Bohemia acknowledged his indebtedness to Wyclif and Martin Luther owed something to the teaching of Huss, so Luther's Protestants were the lineal descendants of Wyclif's Lollards.

There can be little doubt that plague became endemic in Northern

Europe after 1348, erupting into quite large epidemics at frequent intervals. Plague replaced leprosy as the most feared of all diseases. Fear of leprosy had been a revulsion from a horrible but uncommon illness. Fear of plague was entirely justified. The death cart rumbling over the cobbles, the chalked cross on the house door, the useless bonfires in the streets struck terror into men's hearts. Because plague had become endemic, a few cases were ever present as a reminder of the very real danger of widespread epidemic. These major visitations recurred again and again throughout the whole period from 1361 until 1665, sometimes producing a death toll of thousands a week in the crowded walled towns.

One such outbreak in 1635−6 caused about 10,400 deaths in London. This is not a high mortality when compared with 41,300 in 1624 and 68,600 in 1665, but the 1635 plague caused the government of Charles I to take the first known measures to prevent infection. Roughly 1,000 deaths a month occurred from January to April. On 22 April a royal proclamation promulgated rules 'for preventing the spreading of the Plague' and on the same day an Order in Council directed that a rate be levied in the counties of Middlesex and Surrey 'for the erection of Pest Houses and other places of abode for infected persons'. In May the Privy Council complained to the Lord Mayor that crosses were not prominently displayed on doors of infected houses, and that watchmen neglected their duty of keeping people away. In July the Council made orders forbidding Bartholomew Fair, Tutbury Fair, and the well-known fair at Southwark. In October the King ordained a weekly intercessionary fast. This had little effect, for deaths continued throughout the winter and increased in number during spring 1636. At the end of May the inmates of the Fleet Prison petitioned to be allowed to go into the country on parole and their petition was allowed. In June the Council banned all fairs and issued a directive ordering the removal of London children from schools in Enfield, Waltham and 'other towns near his Majesty's house at Theobalds', the stated reason being that parents visited their children and so endangered the King's servants.

The type of rules 'for preventing the spreading of the Plague' are to be found in the minutes of a Common Council meeting at Faversham, Kent. The Council appointed three wardens to examine persons entering the town and refuse admission to anyone coming from a known plague area. They directed all dunghills to be removed and that no new ones be made in or near the town. A woman was appointed to search dead bodies. Her wage was fixed at 11s. a week and she presumably looked for signs of plague. Other common precautions included the notorious red cross and 'Lord Have Mercy on Us' affixed to the doors of infected houses. The patrolling watchmen had the duty, not only of ensuring that the inhabitants remained within, but that passers-by did not loiter in the vicinity. Large fires, kept burning in public places day and night, were often fed with sulphur or other chemicals. The clothing of victims was supposed to be burnt, but relatives generally neglected this very obvious precaution. Specially appointed officers collected bodies for burial in pits, filled with lime, outside the town boundaries. The useless and cruel quarantine, first practised by the town authorities of Ragusa in 1377, will be mentioned in a later chapter.

Regulations at various times ordered the destruction of domestic animals; cats, dogs, pigs. In 1647 a Scottish ordinance directed the laying of poison for rats and mice. At first sight it is remarkable that more attention was not paid to the connection between plague and rodents for, in all modern epidemics such as those of Canton and India, a large mortality of rats has always accompanied or preceded the disease in man. Even in the worst visitations, when the pneumonic form spreads directly from human to human, the rat—flea—man cycle persists and is still the more likely method of dissemination in less highly populated areas. Yet, except for not more than two or three rather doubtful references in ancient texts, no one appears to have noticed the association until after 1894. The reason may be that only wide-scale epidemics attracted public notice. Then the man-to-man transmission, infecting whole households and communities, would have been the more obvious.

Plague virtually disappeared from Northern and Western Europe after 1665. The last great epidemic in Britain was part of a pandemic covering Europe in 1664—5. It is commonly known as the 'Great Plague of London' and has received undue attention partly as being the last and partly because we know more of it than of other plagues from the eye-witness account of Samuel Pepys and Defoe's *Journal*, compiled from second-hand but probably accurate material. This visitation started on 2 November 1664 at Westminster and caused a few deaths throughout the winter. Mortality started to increase at the beginning of June, reaching a peak of about 8,000 a week in September. At the end of September, the number of deaths fell at almost exactly the same angle as the rise, until only a few were recorded in December. In spring 1666 plague recurred, producing about 2,000 deaths during the summer months. The death pattern is very interesting. Contrary to popular belief, the City of London escaped comparatively lightly. The heaviest mortality occurred in the out-parishes of Cripplegate, Whitechapel, Stepney, St Martin-in-the-Fields, St Giles-in-the-Fields, Southwark and Westminster. The plague moved in an arc eastward from Westminster to Stepney, producing maximum mortalities at St Giles in the last week of July, at Cripplegate in the second week of August, and at Stepney in the first three weeks of September. The pattern of death is of some importance because it disproves the 'history book' theory that the 1666 Fire of London put an end to plague. The Fire was almost confined to the City and only touched the worst plague areas at Cripplegate and around Fleet Street. Setting aside the fact that the destruction of London could hardly have affected the course of plague in the rest of England or in Europe, 'purging by fire' of the City cannot have removed foci in the heavily infected out-parishes.

The epidemic died away in England during 1667 and the only recorded deaths from plague for the next 200 years are two cases at Redruth, Cornwall, in 1671. This strange and quite sudden cessation was not confined to Britain; the disease disappeared from the whole of Europe during the eighteen years 1665—83. A new import into Marseilles caused some 50,000 deaths in the city and surrounding countryside in 1720. Another pandemic started in 1855 and moved slowly over Asia, Eastern Europe, and the South Mediterranean seaboard. It arrived at Canton and Hong Kong in May 1894 and caused about 90,000 deaths. Plague was brought by ship to Britain, producing a few cases in Glasgow, one in Cardiff, and eleven in Liverpool during the year 1900—1. Work done during this prolonged and severe outbreak established the method of transmission. On 20 June 1894 Alexandre Yersin, a Swiss bacteriologist practising in Hong Kong, identified *Pasteurella pestis* as the causative organism. Rat mortality had been noted during an Indian epidemic in 1837, but the very large number of dead and dying rats at Canton in 1894 could not possibly escape attention. The same was true at Formosa in 1897, when Ogata Masanori, impressed by the relationship, gave plague the name of 'ratpest'. In Britain, anti-plague measures issued by the Local Government Board in 1900—1 included an order for the destruction of rats and advice that a close watch be kept for evidence of unusual mortality among these pests. Thus, after a lapse of 500 years, the rat was officially recognized as both culprit and victim. The intermediate place of the flea as vector was not fully worked out until 1905.

None of this work explains why plague quite suddenly disappeared from Europe in the seventeenth century. There are a number of theories. One supposes that the port of London provided a focus from which the infection was carried to other parts of the world and that dissemination of shipping to other ports, following the Fire of 1666, reduced the risk. But there is no evidence that London was ever a primary centre; the City appears to have experienced new invasions from abroad rather than distributing plague to foreign countries. A second, rather misty, theory holds that epidemic diseases are a reflection of states of civilization. Leprosy, plague and malaria have all occurred at various times in Britain but are now practically confined to less privileged communities. It is difficult to accept this hypothesis because only a very rash historian would argue that the 'state of civilization' was any higher in a late eighteenth century industrial town than in a seventeenth century city. The Black Rat theory is the most commonly accepted. Black rats and mice are the two rodents which live companionably with man. Further, the black rat is commonly infested with the Indian rat flea, *Xenopsylla cheopis*, which is widely disseminated throughout the world. Unlike the human flea, *Pulex irritans*, the rat flea is a potent vector of plague bacilli, and will forsake the host rat, particularly when dead or dying, for the human. Black rats are known to have been the predominant species in the plague years but are not now common in Europe. Those who support this theory believe that the stronger and more pugnacious Brown or Norwegian rat spread gradually across Europe, killing out the Black rat on its path, and thus destroyed the foci of plague. Here is a reasonable supposition, because the brown rat is not nearly so companionable with man as is the black, and is more commonly infested with a different flea, *Nosopsyllus fasciatus*, which rarely transfers to the human.

Unfortunately this very neat theory takes too much for granted. First, the brown rat did not arrive in Britain until 1728, over sixty years after the last great epidemic, and the black was still the predominant species in London until after 1783. Second, the black rat reappeared in London about 1911 and by 1937 outnumbered the brown as a town-rat. Third, the suggestion that black rats were killed out by more ferocious brown rats is a mere assumption. The two kinds seem to live more or less in amity.

A curious incident, sometimes known as the Black Death of Suffolk, may throw light on the problem. Between 9 December 1906 and 16 June 1918, twenty-one people fell ill of a mysterious disease in a very small area near the mouth of the River Orwell. Sixteen of the twenty-one patients died. Fourteen people suffered from a very virulent pneumonia and seven from an illness described by one of the survivors as 'headache, sickness, diarrhoea, sores, and knots in the neck and groin'. The cases were distributed between five cottages, all of them remote from large population centres.

One of the victims, a nine-year-old child named Anne Goodall, living at Latimer Cottages in the parish of Freston, fell ill of pneumonia on 13 September 1910. She died on 16 September. Her mother, her step-father Mr Chapman, and a woman who nursed the step-father all died of pneumonia within a fortnight. Specimens of blood from Mrs Chapman and of fluid from Mr Chapman's lungs were taken by Dr Llewellyn Heath, a bacteriologist, who grew from them bacilli which he identified as *Pasteurella pestis*. The Local Government Board inspector, Dr Bulstrode, was then called in and sent Heath's specimens to the Board's bacteriological adviser, Dr Klein, who denied the identification of *P. pestis*. However, ten days later Klein received a rat and a hare from the neighbourhood and found both to be infected with plague bacilli. Shortly afterwards he was sent other specimens of rodents from the same district and identified the plague bacillus in these. Dr Bulstrode therefore instigated a programme of rat destruction and laboratory examination.

This investigation produced some interesting evidence. The first large-scale extermination took place in the winter of 1910—11. No plague bacilli were discovered in the 6,071 rats examined. At the same time, flea infestation was investigated; a second batch of 568 rats yielded 584 fleas, 324 being of types which bite man. Of the flea-infested rats, seventeen were found to be infected with plague bacilli. In another parish, Hollesley, workers found three infected rats and two rabbits out of forty examined. The next search took place in the hot weather months July to October 1911. Of 15,332 rodents collected from 27 parishes there were 35 infected rats. The flea population averaged four per rat (i.e. about four times the winter figure) and 60 per cent were of a type which bites the human. In 1913 three parishes harboured infected rats and seven infected ferrets were also discovered. Four rats and one rabbit, similarly infected, were found in

1914; the investigation ended with the outbreak of war. During the whole of this research, only one black rat was discovered in the urban area of Ipswich. All other rats were of the brown kind.

Although infection of rodents by the plague bacillus had been demonstrated, the human diagnosis was doubtful. In October 1911 a sailor stationed at the Royal Naval Barracks, Shotley, became ill after sustaining a small cut while cleaning a rabbit which he had caught near Latimer Cottages, Freston. The diagnosis of plague is said to have been confirmed by examination of the sputum, but the history is so suggestive of septicaemia that the present writer has not included the sailor among the twenty-one cases. No such doubt attaches to the final cases of Mrs Bugg and her next door neighbour, Mrs Garrod, who lived at Warren Lane Cottages, Ewarton, a mile from Shotley Barracks. Both died of a virulent pneumonia in June 1918. Sputum from Mrs Garrod, examined by Captain Cade, RAMC, bacteriologist to the Eastern Command, revealed *Pasteurella pestis*.

It is certain that this prolonged and disparate epidemic was plague, for similar incidents have occurred in other parts of the world. The plague is of a type known as 'campestral' or 'sylvatic', a disease of wild rodents, such as rats, rabbits, hares, squirrels. Rodent—flea—rodent transmission can carry infection to the more urban or companionable type of animal, black rats, hamsters, guinea pigs. When this occurs there is risk to the human and, indeed, risk of a large epidemic. But, very rarely, the sylvatic type may be transmitted to the human without the intermediate domestic animal. This will happen if a human is bitten by a flea from an infected wild rodent or if he happens to cut himself when the animal is in contact with his skin. Consideration of the figures given on (p. 72) will show that the risk is very small. Among 15,332 rodents collected in the hot weather months, when activity is greatest, only 35 were infected. These 35 bore 140 fleas, nearly half of which were of types which do not infest the human. But the disease produced is plague and carries a very high mortality.

The Suffolk epidemic is characterized by a number of small outbreaks in scattered, isolated houses. When attacked, the whole family became ill and most of them died. In one case eight people, four of them in one family, fell ill and six died, the maximum length of illness being five days. In another, seven members of a family named Rouse, living in an overcrowded cottage, fell sick. Four died and three recovered. Taking into consideration the rarity of infected rodents, it is quite inconceivable that each separate member of the family was bitten by an individual flea from an infected animal. It is equally inconceivable that a single flea hopped from member to member. We are left with the fair certainty that, after the initial infection of one member of the family, plague was transmitted to the others either by direct human-to-human or by the human—flea—human route. In other words, the rodent played no further part after the initial infection.

Here is a possible explanation of the explosive pandemic in 1348, the later widespread epidemics, and the disappearance of plague after 1671. The epidemiology as described in previous pages is correct but operated in reverse. Our forefathers, who were just as observant as we are, failed to notice a high mortality among rats because no such mortality occurred. During the early years of European plague, the black rat played no part in its spread. Europe had not experienced the disease for 800 years, and the people were in consequence entirely unprotected. Plague was a human disease, transmitted either directly man-to-man or by man—flea—man, the former method being the more probable. At some time during the next three centuries *Pasteurella pestis* developed a predilection for the companionable black rat, probably a reversion to its previous host in Central Asia, being carried to the rat by the type of flea common to both rats and men. The plague caused a continual diminution of rats which had little or no relation to epidemics among humans. But the death of so many rats also caused a very great decrease in the number of rat fleas, since the flea can only exist on the living rat. The critical time came in 1665—83 when only the human host remained in sufficient numbers to ensure the continuance of plague. No human epidemic in fact developed and the process of flea and rat attrition went on for almost 100 years until the black rat was virtually exterminated in Europe. In the end plague, in the form of sylvatic plague, only existed among such wild species as had acquired it by casual contact with the original hosts.

Whatever the answer may be, and the above is supposition only, the 300 years reign of plague ended by some natural process and not by any active measures on the part of men. There is no medical or scientific discovery, no advance in social hygiene, no improved standard of life, which can possibly account for its disappearance. Plague ended—or went into hiding. For we must always remember that three plague-free centuries separate us from 1665, and eight plague-free centuries separated the Plague of Justinian from the Black Death.

5   Prevention of smallpox

After plague disappeared in the mid-seventeenth century, smallpox took its place as the most dreaded of all diseases. This does not imply that smallpox was unknown before 1665. Gregory of Tours described an epidemic in AD 581, and in 1314 an English physician, John of Gaddesden, advised hangings of red cloth as part of treatment, a method similar to that of Niels Finsen in 1893, using red light. But it is difficult to disentangle the early history of smallpox from that of several other diseases. The difficulty is partly one of nomenclature. A quite common sixteenth century diagnosis is 'smallpoxe and mesles' applied to a single illness. From the beginning of the sixteenth century, 'great pox' indicated the major cutaneous eruption of syphilis and probably other severe skin diseases. Smallpox seems to have been used for lesser eruptions, a collection of ailments characterized by a rash, such as chicken pox, measles, smallpox and secondary syphilis.

These are known as acute infections or sometimes as zymotic diseases. They are illnesses of the crowd and cannot have flourished among the small, scattered settlements of primitive man. Their origin lies in the early large concentrations of the human race, such as the Nile Valley, Mesopotamia, India and China. The causative organism of an acute infection can only transfer from one person to another when the disease is active, that is other people can only acquire measles from a person who is actually suffering from measles. The method of transmission differs from that of typhoid fever, carried by infected water, or bubonic plague which can be carried by a flea from an infected animal.

One attack of an acute infection will confer upon the sufferer immunity from further attacks. Immunity may be short lived or sometimes for life. A fully immune individual cannot acquire the disease or transmit it. The infection is never entirely absent from the community but requires a reservoir of people who have never suffered the disease to ensure continuity. The number of susceptible children will be at a minimum after a severe and widespread epidemic of measles. Measles then occurs only sporadically until there is a new generation of susceptible children. When the number of susceptible children forms a substantial part of the community, the chance of transmission from a sporadic case will be high and so another large scale epidemic will occur.

Measles confers a long-lived immunity and, until a few years ago, was so common that few Europeans reached adult life without suffering an attack. Thus, European measles was a true 'childish disease'. But if measles is introduced into a community which has never before experienced the infection, all age groups will be at risk. Further, a limited maternal immunity is conferred upon the child. Such maternal immunity may not be sufficient to prevent an attack, but the illness will not usually be of a severe type. Since an unaccustomed group possess no immunity, hereditary or acquired, they will suffer the full effect. This is why a new disease may be so lethal that it is barely recognizable as the form existing in a community which has experienced it for many years.

Historically, the large epidemics of childish disease have been of economic importance in social development. When the disease has been a lethal one, such as is smallpox or infantile diarrhoea, recurrent epidemics with a high mortality have prevented a too rapid increase in child population. A poverty-stricken people, breeding without check, will produce families of a size which the wage-earning parents cannot support. Less than two centuries ago expectation of life was short and the older non-productive age group posed no problem. But the younger unproductive element might have reached such a proportion that it could not be fed by the productive. There is little doubt that this state would have come to pass had it not been for the natural check imposed by a high disease mortality in infancy and early childhood.

Smallpox exists in three forms. *Variola major* is true virulent smallpox; *Variola minor* or alastrim is a comparatively mild illness; *Variola vaccinae* is cowpox, a disease of animals which can be transmitted to the human. An attack of any one form will protect, at least temporarily, against the other two. The question is—which form was prevalent in Western Europe before the end of the seventeenth century? In 1901 Paul Kübler made the pertinent observation that *Variola major* can hardly have existed in the Greek or Roman civilizations, because there is no known classical statue or caricature which portrays a pock mark and no mention of any such disfigurement by medical or lay authors. The typical and persistent pock mark, which often appears in eighteenth and nineteenth century literature, can hardly have escaped notice. Rhazes describes pock marks about AD 900 in his book on smallpox and measles, but he was writing of the disease in the Near and Middle East. Even Rhazes implies in one passage that measles is a more malignant illness than smallpox.

There is no record during the Dark Ages or mediaeval period of a violent epidemic, attacking all age groups and carrying a high mortality, followed by lesser but still virulent outbreaks which we could identify as the first invasion of smallpox. Yet smallpox did exist in Western Europe from at least as early as AD 580, but it does not seem to have been regarded as a very serious disease. We must conclude that the smallpox of the Middle Ages was the mild alastrim, probably occurring as a childish illness, causing an appreciable number of deaths, and occasionally erupting into epidemics. As a general rule, it must have been a not very dangerous feverish illness with an accompanying rash. Since the treatment of any such illness would have been the same, exact diagnosis did not matter. Doctors were rarely called in to advise on childish ailments; even in wealthy families, the care of a sick child devolved upon the nurse. The majority of children were tended by their parents, sometimes advised by a wise-woman or midwife. A diagnosis of 'The poor child's got the pox and fever' would be more likely than an attempt to differentiate between smallpox, measles or chicken pox, a distinction which could have made not the slightest difference to the treatment or fate of the patient.

But European smallpox undoubtedly changed its character, presumably because the lethal *Variola major* replaced the mild alastrim. The change took place gradually and not by means of a sudden and violent epidemic. This insidious alteration in the nature of the disease is explicable if we allow that a large proportion of the population was already protected by an attack of alastrim. It is much more difficult to explain why the change occurred. There is known to be some mutation which can alter the nature of a microorganism, just as genetic mutation effects alteration in the human. An instance is the penicillin-resistant strain which has developed from a mutant, adapting itself to survive the ability of penicillin to reduce the microorganism's reproductive power. Mutation may explain the change but, equally, it could have been brought about by European contact with an exotic and more lethal virus. The time at which *Variola major* emerged as a severe and widespread illness suggests that the latter reason is the more likely.

There are several possible sources. As mentioned in the last chapter (p. 61), the fifteenth and sixteenth centuries witnessed a search for the sea route to the East, either by passage round the Cape of Good Hope or by the western approach deemed possible through ignorance that America stood in the way. Virulent smallpox existed in China, being described by the physician Ko Hung who lived AD 265—313. Ralph Major holds alastrim to have been the prevalent form in India until the sixteenth century, when *Variola major* appeared as an import from China. Here is a possible source, for a limited European contact with India existed after Vasco da Gama landed at Calicut on 20 May 1498. Tropical Africa, where smallpox was very prevalent, must also be considered, but we know little of the history of disease in this area and must regard it as equally probable that Europeans introduced the lethal form into an unprotected community.

An ingenious and quite plausible theory depends upon the 'refreshment' of an old and less virulent strain by introduction into a community which has never previously experienced any form of the disease. There is no doubt that the expeditions led by Hernando Cortez and Panfilo de Narvaez carried smallpox into Central America between the years 1518 and 1520. When Mexico City fell to Cortez in August 1521, the Spaniards found houses filled with dead. The epidemic spread rapidly; within six months hardly one village in the known regions of New Spain remained uninfected. Mortality was quite appalling. It has been estimated that nearly half the native population died in this first epidemic. The theory depends upon the supposition that the Conquistadores introduced alastrim to the unprotected Central American Indians in whom it produced a lethal illness, which was returned to Europe. But the story is not clear. According to one account, Narvaez carried a number of African slaves on his voyage from Cuba to Mexico in May 1520. Some of these fell ill on board ship, at least one being landed while still sick. Since King Ferdinand of Spain first sent African slaves to the West Indies in 1502, it is possible that the initial infection came from Africa.

Whether by 'refreshment' of an old strain or by introduction of a new, Variola major appeared in Europe during the sixteenth century and seems to have become fairly common in Britain by the time of James I. The two forms, major and minor, existed side by side. The minor remained a childish disease, the major tended to attack older children and adults. Variola major seems to have been gradually 'taking over' from the mild alastrim throughout the seventeenth century. The London Bills of Mortality are notoriously inaccurate and cannot be regarded as of statistical value, but they do reveal broad trends in the rise and decline of various diseases for the two centuries from 1629 until 1837, the first year of death registration. The Bills show a gradual rise in smallpox deaths throughout the seventeenth century. The peak year was 1681 and then came a fall until 1710. The fall was interrupted by quite large epidemics in 1685 and 1694–5, one of the victims of the latter being Queen Mary. Without placing too much reliance on the Bills, we may say that the death rate throughout the century varied between 250 and 2,500 per year in a population of about 400,000. Nearly 3,000 people are recorded as having died in the 1681 epidemic and just over 2,000 in 1685.

A change in the age incidence started at the beginning of the eighteenth century. Variola major became the most common and most lethal disease of young children. The change was general throughout Europe and, although not easy to understand, must be connected with a preponderance of the 'major strain' over the 'minor strain'. It is probably true to say that alastrim disappeared, to be replaced by severe or less severe attacks of Variola major. The Bills of Mortality now show an annual death rate of around 2,000, only five years in which deaths were under 1,000 and eleven in which deaths exceeded 3,000. About 80 per cent of these deaths were in children under five years old. In one English town, 589 children died of smallpox between 1769 and 1774. Of these, 466 were under three years old and only one over ten. The rest of Europe showed a similar pattern. At about the same period, 98 per cent of all deaths from smallpox in Berlin were of children below the age of twelve. The contemporary physician Rosen von Rosenstein stated that smallpox every year killed one-tenth of all Swedish children in their first year of life. With the possible exception of infantile diarrhoea, smallpox had become the greatest natural check upon an uncontrolled rise in population.

During the eighteenth century smallpox became particularly prevalent in the expanding industrial towns, a development only to be expected as it is one of the more infectious diseases. Towns continued to grow at an even more rapid rate throughout the nineteenth century but the incidence and death rate of smallpox both declined. Decline in London started about 1796. The Bills of Mortality now show a steep fall in deaths from 3,500 in 1796 to a yearly average of about 800 in the two decades 1810–30. From 1838, the first full year of registration, we have reliable statistics for the whole of England and Wales. These figures show a remarkable decrease throughout the nineteenth century, from 16,268 deaths in 1838 to 20 in 1899. The graph of this steady fall is broken by a major epidemic which caused just over 23,000 deaths in 1871 and 19,000 in 1872.

The high mortality for 1838 is attributable to an epidemic lasting from 1837 until 1840. Between 1840 and 1871 six smaller epidemics occurred which each produced 300–400 deaths, roughly double the annual average for the rest of the period. From 1872 until 1899 there were four epidemics, none of which caused more than 150 deaths, about three times the average mortality of other years. Both sporadic and epidemic smallpox tended to be localized, a disease of cities and of the London slums in particular. The age distribution also changed. Of the total smallpox deaths in London, the percentage occurring in the first five years of life fell from the eighteenth century 80 per cent to 62 per cent in 1851–60, 54 per cent in 1861–70 and 30 per cent in 1871–80. Charles Creighton, a leading historian of English epidemic disease, sums up the eighteenth and nineteenth century decline of smallpox 'It first left the richer classes, then it left the villages, then it left the provincial towns, to centre itself in the capital; at the same time it was leaving the age of infancy and childhood.'

British smallpox remained one of the major killers for rather less than a century. Case mortality never approached that of plague; although incidence was high, many patients recovered. A person who survived an attack was usually marked for life. The stigma reminded a healthy man that he too is mortal, and partly explains the peculiar horror which smallpox aroused. The pock mark also set a fashion. The elegant eighteenth century, 'the age of powder and patches' is the time when the pock mark was most common and acquired in early life. The strange 'beauty patch', a scrap of coloured material which appears in so many portraits, was utilitarian in origin, designed to hide a skin blemish.

Attempts have been made to prevent disease from time immemorial. They have taken various forms such as sacrifice, votive offerings, or self-flagellation. The doctrine of signatures, resemblance of the offered sacrifice to the object desired, suggested that certain ills might be warded off by similar materials; a tooth-shaped stone to prevent toothache is the simple example. Talismans were sacred or magical words written on parchment; amulets, a motley array of strange objects. These guarded not only against ill-luck but against disease. There are people today who believe that a potato carried in the pocket will prevent rheumatism. The potato is probably an amulet rather than a prophylactic. Then there is a part of the diseased beast or human. The hair of the dog was not originally an alcoholic drink to cure an alcoholic hangover, but the actual hair of a rabid dog laid on the bite or swallowed to avert hydrophobia.

This last belief probably induced the first attempts to prevent smallpox. About AD 1000 Chinese physicians collected scales from drying smallpox pustules, ground them to powder, and blew a few grains into the nostrils of the person to be protected. Another method of protection derived from the knowledge that some illnesses are by nature chronic and some acute, that a patient may fall sick of the same disease quite often and that other diseases will attack only once in a lifetime. The phenomenon of acquired immunity, though not expressed, must have been observed. Reason would suggest that if a dangerous disease does not strike a person more than once, a mild attack of that disease is wholly desirable. It would then be reasonable to suppose that an individual might be protected by placing him in contact with the mildest form available. We know that this was often done.

Perhaps the best known instance is that recorded by John Evelyn in his *Diary*. The year of 1685 was a bad one for Evelyn. He lost two daughters from smallpox within six months. The younger, Mary, was nineteen years old. Mr Hussey, a young man in love with Mary, died the same year and of the same disease. On 13 September 1685 Evelyn travelled with Samuel Pepys to Portsmouth. After dinner on the first day they hired a coach and drove to Bagshot, arriving in time for supper.

> Whilst supper was making ready, I went and made a visit to Mrs Graham, sometime Maid of Honour to the Queene Dowager, now wife to James Graham, Esq., of the privy purse to the King. . . . Her eldest son was now sick there of the small-pox, but in a likely way to recovery, and other of her children ran about and among the infected, which she said she let them do on purpose that they might whilst young pass that fatal disease she fancied they were to undergo one time or other, and that this would be for the best: the severity of this cruell disease so lately in my poore family confirming much of what she affirmed.

A combination of the folk belief that like cures or prevents like with this crude method of purposeful contact suggested a refinement, transplantation of tissue or secretion from a mildly affected patient into the person to be protected. At the beginning of the eighteenth century a Greek physician practising in Smyrna, Giacomo Pylarini, removed some of the thick matter from a pustule and rubbed it into a small scratch made with a needle. Another Greek, Emanuel Timoni of Constantinople, adopted his method and sent an account to Dr John Woodward of London. Woodward described the work of Pylarini and Timoni at a meeting of the Royal Society, the report being published in *Philosophical Transactions* in 1714. This method is inoculation which, in view of later developments, is better described as *variolation* or the inoculation of the actual matter of smallpox.

Three years later Lady Mary Wortley Montagu, wife of the British ambassador in Constantinople, returned to England, having already had her infant son inoculated in that city. In 1721 a quite severe epidemic of smallpox, causing some 3,000 deaths, occurred in London. Lady Mary had her five-year-old daughter inoculated in the presence of several physicians who were much impressed by the mildness of the subsequent attack. The physicians received royal permission to make a trial. Six prisoners under sentence of death at Newgate Prison volunteered on the promise of a reprieve. The physicians made a second trial on eleven charity school children of varying ages. In every case the resulting attack was so mild that George I commanded variolation of two grandchildren.

The entire credit for the introduction of variolation into England has been given to Lady Mary Wortley Montagu, but there is no doubt the credit is undeserved. Woodward's communication to the Royal Society exercised far greater influence. Lady Mary's enthusiasm lent the method a certain atmosphere of aristocratic approval. There followed a short-lived fashion for variolation in Britain, Europe and America, where the famous Puritan divine, Cotton Mather, became an ardent advocate. It is significant that Mather was a Fellow of the Royal Society. But variolation is inoculation with smallpox. The ensuing and protecting attack did not always take a mild course; it has been reckoned that, in this first phase, 2 or 3 deaths occurred in every 100 inoculations. Further, without rigid segregation of the subject, variolation spread disease. These dangers soon came to be recognized and the method was rarely practised in Britain and Europe after 1728.

Events took a different turn in the American colonies, where smallpox had been introduced into Maryland by British settlers during the last years of the seventeenth century. A big epidemic, possibly an offshoot of the English outbreak, came from the West Indies in 1721. Cotton Mather suggested a large scale trial of variolation. Only one physician, Zabdiel Boylston, showed interest. By September 1721 he had inoculated thirty-five people with satisfactory results and no deaths. Despite this success Boylston was accused of spreading smallpox and narrowly escaped lynching. In 1738 a severe epidemic ravaged the town of Charleston, South Carolina. Dr James Kilpatrick carried out a programme of mass variolation and claimed that a high mortality had thereby been prevented. At about this time Benjamin Franklin lost his only son from smallpox and became a fervent advocate of variolation. It may have been Franklin who later influenced George Washington. During the War of Independence Washington urged inoculation on his troops and set up special hospitals for the purpose.

Dr James Kilpatrick came to London from Charleston in 1743. He wrote an account of the 1738 epidemic and emphasized the usefulness of variolation. Kilpatrick also described an 'improved method'. Previous inoculators had believed that the method would be useless unless the 'variolous matter' was inserted deeply in the layer of fat beneath the skin. Kilpatrick insisted on a very shallow scratch, which tended to produce a local rather than a general infection. Through his enthusiasm and because of a greatly increased incidence of smallpox, variolation came back into fashion in the second half of the eighteenth century. In 1747 Richard Mead, one of the most influential physicians of his day, published a book in which he strongly supported the practice.

'Inoculators' were specialists in the art and often not medically qualified. Some of the more famous names are Robert Sutton, his son Daniel, Jan IngenHousz and Thomas Dimsdale. The Suttons developed the method of 'removes'. They took the mildest available case of smallpox, inoculated perhaps a dozen people therefrom, again chose the mildest case and so on. When a VIP was to be the subject, the inoculator used a number of removes. IngenHousz, who treated the Austrian court in 1768, inoculated over 200 individuals, probably ten or more removes. Voltaire became a firm believer in variolation and he is supposed to have aroused the interest of the Russian Empress, Catherine the Great, thus initiating one of the more famous incidents in the history of preventive medicine. In 1768 Catherine invited Thomas Dimsdale to visit St Petersburg where, after inoculating a number of servants, he treated the Empress, her son Paul, and members of the imperial court. Dimsdale received a fee of £10,000, an additional £2,000 for expenses, an annuity of £500, diamond studded miniatures of Catherine and her son, and the rank of Baron.

Many inoculators, having passaged the lymph through several removes, used the end product on a number of people and over a considerable period of time. This practice increased the risk of transmitting extraneous infection. Edward Jenner writes that

> a medical gentleman (now no more) who inoculated great numbers in this neighbourhood, frequently preserved his matter on a piece of Lint or Cotton which, in its wet state, was put into a vial, corked up, and convey'd into a warm Pocket, a situation certainly favourable for producing putrefaction in it. In this state (not unfrequently after it had been taken several days from the pustules) it was inserted into the arms of his Patients, and brought on inflammation in the incised parts, swellings of the Axillary Glands, fever, and (as I have been inform'd by the Patients themselves) eruptions.

Here is a clear indication that people were inoculated with pathogenic organisms other than the smallpox virus. Illness and even death must have been quite common. Inoculators claimed that their improved methods had reduced the 1721—8 mortality of 2—3 in every 100 to 1 per 1,000. It is very unlikely that mortality even fell to so low a figure.

Whatever the death rate, there is no doubt that variolation often failed to give protection. Many inoculators believed that the severity of the subsequent illness depended upon the depth at which the lymph was inserted. Trying to produce the mildest possible attack, they made only a superficial scratch on the skin which produced no reaction, general or local. Since a certain magic always attaches to a procedure like inoculation, it must have been quite common for people to believe themselves protected when they were not. The consequent disappointment would have dispelled confidence in the efficacy of variolation. Further, if successful, the risk of spreading smallpox remained. The danger was widely recognized. Many practitioners maintained isolation houses in which their patients could stay until free of infection. Several physicians advised the foundation of inoculation hospitals where the poor might be treated. One of these, the London Smallpox and Inoculation Hospital, founded in 1746, profoundly influenced later events.

Some medical historians believe that variolation almost ceased to be used in the last years of the eighteenth century because not only doctors but the public recognized that the practice was neither safe nor efficient. This is not true. The poor-house account books of a small Somerset village provide an example:

> May ye 21st 1769. It is this day agreed upon by the churchwardens and overseers and the other inhabitants of the said Parish of Fitzhead that all poor children that have been chargeable to the said parish, at a parish meeting held this day or a Vestry for that purpose held, shall be inoculated by the parish expence, as Witness our hands John Comer, John Arscott, Jno. Holcombe, William Toogood.

1769	Paid for inoculating of the parish	01.15.00
1789	Paid Dr Comer his bill for inoculating 27 poor people, due last year	05.08.00
1796	Paid Mr Sully for inocklating Thirty Four children	08.10.00
1798	Towards Inocklating Stook and Stones children	00.15.00
1798	Paid for inocklating Wm Crewse three children	00.07.06

Right at the end of its history, variolation must have been used extensively and by no means only for the wealthier class.*

A new method of protection was suggested in 1798. Again, this depended upon chance observation and not upon knowledge of the cause. Folk medicine quite frequently, and often rightly, holds that people who work in certain trades are particularly susceptible to certain ailments, while people working in other trades are unusually immune. Knowledge that miners are prone to suffer from diseases of the lung was widespread in the sixteenth century. Doctors confirmed the folk belief that butchers rarely suffered from consumption. There is an old tradition, very prevalent in the West Country, that farm hands who work with cattle are never attacked by smallpox. No one knows who stumbled on the truth that it is not cattle, but a disease of cattle, which protects. The lesions of cowpox must have been often observed on the hands of dairymaids.

Cowpox or *Variola vaccinae* is not a common disease but, once introduced into a herd, may infect a number of beasts. It usually appears

---

* P. E. Razzell ('Population Change in 18th century England', in M. Drahe (edit.), *Population in Industrialization*, London, 1969, pp. 128—56) draws attention to the wide prevalence of variolation, often with some measure of compulsion, in the second half of the eighteenth century. Razzell propounds the theory that variolation so decreased mortality from smallpox as to be a significant factor in the massive rise of population.

upon the udder and, unless quickly treated, will produce ulcers which affect the cow's health and diminish milk secretion. Treatment was fairly easy even in the eighteenth century; applications of sulphate of zinc or copper were effective. The lesion is very contagious. A person who milks an infected cow is liable to develop cowpox on the hands or wrists. The risk of man-to-man spread is slight. Only very rarely is the skin lesion followed by a generalized illness, although there is often slight fever and malaise. Transmission is by direct contact; matter from the ulcer must impinge upon a scratch in the skin before a human can acquire the disease.

Since cowpox is uncommon, we need not wonder that its power to protect against smallpox remained little more than a fable. One deliberate attempt is known to have been made but it had no influence upon the future history. In 1774 an epidemic of smallpox visited Dorset. Benjamin Jesty, a farmer of Yetminster near Yeovil, being aware of the cowpox fable, allowed two farm hands, who had both suffered from the disease, to nurse smallpox patients. Both remained uninfected. Shortly afterwards, Jesty found one of his cows to be suffering. He took matter from a lesion and rubbed it into scratches made with a darning needle on the arms of his wife and two sons. None of them acquired smallpox, but Jesty was strongly criticized for his inhuman experiment. Fifteen years later, in 1789, a doctor named Trowbridge, practising in the near-by village of Cerne Abbas, must have heard of the incident. He got in touch with Jesty's sons and persuaded them to let him inoculate them with smallpox. No reaction followed, either local or general. Trowbridge forfeited his chance of fame by failing to do any more work. Possibly he could find no one else who had suffered from cowpox in his district.

Edward Jenner, born at Berkeley in Gloucestershire on 17 May 1749, served an apprenticeship at Sodbury and then as a house pupil to the great surgeon John Hunter at St George's Hospital, London. Both men loved natural history, a bond which resulted in a firm friendship lasting from 1770 until Hunter's death in 1793. In 1772 Jenner set up in practice at Berkeley, where he found plenty of time for study and to undertake investigations suggested by Hunter. His original work earned him election to the Royal Society in 1789. Hunter's most famous dictum 'but why think, why not try the experiment?' is contained in a letter to Jenner on the subject of hedgehogs.

'Why think, why not try the experiment?' Although written by John Hunter, the words might serve as a title for Jenner's biography. It is common knowledge that Edward Jenner inoculated the boy James Phipps with cowpox matter taken from the hand of a dairymaid, Sarah Nelmes, in 1796. It is not so commonly understood that this was no isolated incident, no trial suggested by chance observation, but the culminating point of an investigation when only human experiment could prove a theory which had occupied Jenner's mind for twenty years. The cowpox story first came to his attention in the 1770s when an apprentice to Daniel Ludlow, a surgeon of Sodbury. A milkmaid told Jenner 'I cannot take smallpox for I have had cowpox.' He later passed this piece of information on to John Hunter, who mentioned it as a traditional belief in his lectures.

In 1778, when he was practising at Berkeley 'Mrs H. a respectable Gentlewoman of this town' consulted Jenner. Smallpox was rife in Berkeley at the time. Mrs H. had suffered from cowpox, apparently communicated from a human source. Later she had nursed a relative suffering from smallpox without catching it. Mrs H. wanted to know whether she could consider herself safe or whether she ought to be inoculated. Jenner saw his opportunity, inoculated her from a smallpox pustule and observed a slight local reaction but no other sign of illness. Between 1791 and 1795 he found several people who had suffered from cowpox and inoculated them with similar results. One of these was a woman who had had cowpox in 1760. Jenner inoculated her in 1791 and she subsequently nursed several smallpox patients without ill effect. It may be this case, with its thirty year lapse between cowpox infection and variolation, which gave Jenner the wrong impression that cowpox protects for life.

In May 1796 an outbreak of cowpox occurred on two dairy farms near Berkeley. Jenner, now reasonably certain that the traditional belief was correct, decided on the crucial test.

> The more accurately to observe the progress of the infection, I selected a healthy boy about eight years old for the purpose of inoculation with the cowpox. The matter was taken from a suppurated sore on the hand of a dairy Maid who was infected by her master's Cows, and it was inserted on the 14th of May 1796, into the arms of the Boy, by means of two superficial incisions, each about three quarters of an inch long. On the 7th day he complained of uneasiness in the Axilla, and on the 9th he became a little chilly, lost his appetite and had a slight headache. During the whole of this day he was perceptibly indisposed, and had rather a restless night; but, on the day following, he was perfectly well. The appearance, and progress of the incisions to a state of maturation, were pretty much the same as when produced in a similar manner by variolous matter. The only difference which I perceived, was, that the edges assumed rather a darker hue, and that the efflorescence spreading round the incisions, took on rather more of an erysipelatous look, than we commonly perceive when variolous matter has been made use of for the same purpose.
>
> On the 1st of July following this Boy was inoculated with Matter immediately taken from a smallpox Pustule. Several punctures and slight incisions were made in both his arms, and the matter was well rubb'd into them, but no disease follow'd. The same appearances only were observable on the arms, as when a Patient has had variolous matter applied, after having either the Cow-pox or the Small pox.

The above account of the vaccination of James Phipps is taken from Jenner's unpublished *On the Cow Pox. The original Paper*. He had satisfied himself that inoculation with *Variola vaccinae* would protect against smallpox, but realized that his professional colleagues would not be satisfied with one successful case. He decided to defer publication until he had more evidence. Unfortunately cowpox disappeared from the neighbourhood of Berkeley in 1796 and did not return until 1798. Unable to find active lesions for further experiments, Jenner investigated the two outbreaks of cowpox which had recently occurred. He found that the first farm employed five people. All except one dairymaid had suffered from smallpox. The farmer and a boy escaped infection with cowpox entirely. Two more workers developed nothing but a small 'sore' on one finger. The dairymaid who had not suffered smallpox 'caught the complaint from the cows and was affected with it in so violent a degree that she was incapable of doing any work for the space of ten days'. In March 1797 Jenner checked by inoculating her with smallpox, and she showed no reaction. On the second farm the staff consisted of the farmer, his wife, two sons, a man and a dairymaid. All, except the farmer, helped in the milking and all, except the man, had suffered from smallpox. The whole staff developed cowpox lesions, but the man was the only one to be severely affected. Jenner inoculated him with matter from a smallpox pustule in February 1797 without any effect. He now had evidence of the reverse postulate, that smallpox will protect against cowpox.

Cowpox recurred in 1798 and Jenner resumed his experiments with matter obtained from active lesions. He 'vaccinated' twenty-three subjects, inoculating them with smallpox after a lapse of some weeks. In every case, inoculation failed to produce anything but a very minor local reaction. In the same year Jenner published his great classic, a seventy-five page pamphlet entitled *An Enquiry into the Causes and Effects of the Variola Vaccinae, a Disease discovered in some of the Western Counties of England, particularly Gloucestershire, and known by the name of Cow Pox.* Jenner had carefully thought out his subject and had conducted experiments as opportunity offered over a number of years. He did not put his theory to the crucial test until he had good reason to believe that no harm would result. He did not rush into print. Even with an assured success and although frustrated by the absence of cowpox, he resisted the temptation to publish his findings until he had proved them beyond question. Jenner was a true scientist.

His paper had a mixed reception by both doctors and public. The inoculators obviously attacked Jenner's vaccination, because its general adoption would end their lucrative trade. His method became a favoured subject for cartoonists. James Gillray depicted an unconcerned doctor vaccinating his patients, surrounded by a terrified crowd with cow's heads appearing from various parts of their bodies and horns bursting from their foreheads. Clergy thundered from the pulpit against the iniquity of transferring disease from the beasts of the field to Man. The protests of those who objected that other and worse infections might be transmitted from cattle to the human were more rational. This last criticism, combined with a rather natural distaste for inoculation with matter from a sick cow, induced early vaccinators to adopt an arm-to-arm technique whenever possible. It became customary to perform one inoculation with cowpox from the animal and then to set up a chain by vaccinating from one human to another. The method proved successful and disposed of the objection to 'animal matter' but added considerably to the danger of transmitting diseases such as syphilis.

The ravages of smallpox were so fearful and variolation had done so little to check epidemics that vaccination rapidly became popular. Doctors soon recognized that cowpox could not be spread except by direct contact and that smallpox never followed. Thus the great objection that variolation might protect the individual but helped to spread the disease did not apply to vaccination. Henry Cline, a leading surgeon of Guy's Hospital, repeated Jenner's experiments and reported favourably. John Coakley Lettsom, a physician who had strongly advocated inoculation hospitals, now came out in support of vaccination. Dr William Woodville of the London Smallpox and Inoculation Hospital, and Dr George Pearson of St George's were other influential men who became enthusiasts.

About 100,000 people had been vaccinated in Britain by the end of 1801 and the method was rapidly coming into worldwide use. It now became difficult to provide sufficient active vaccine and quite extraordinary methods were sometimes adopted. Many people sent matter from the cowpox pustule on threads or porcelain-tipped probes, but the virus lost potency on a long journey. In 1803 the King of Spain decided to introduce vaccination into his American colonies. Twenty-two children who had never suffered from smallpox were enlisted and two of these vaccinated. On the voyage, two fresh children were vaccinated every ten days from the arms of the previous pair. Thus the living vaccine arrived at the port of Caracas. Here the expedition split into two, one part going to South America, where over 50,000 people were vaccinated in Peru alone. The second ship picked up twenty-six fresh children and carried the chain round the world to the Philippines, Macao and Canton. British and American missionaries took vaccine into the Chinese interior.

Almost more romantic is the story of how vaccine reached India, one of the areas most ravaged by smallpox. Jenner advised using a series of children but the Secretary of State, Lord Hobart, would not give permission. The British made several attempts to send vaccine in containers but it proved useless on arrival. At the end of 1801 Mr and Mrs W. H. Nisbet visited their son-in-law Lord Elgin, ambassador at Constantinople. While travelling across Europe, the Nisbets saw Dr Jean de Carro of Vienna performing vaccinations with lymph sent by Dr George Pearson of London. They found smallpox to be rife in Constantinople and persuaded Lord Elgin to send to Vienna for lymph. De Carro dispatched a small supply in a quill, packed in a glass bottle. With this, Lord Elgin himself vaccinated his eighteen-month-old son. The child's arm supplied enough lymph to vaccinate members of the Diplomatic Corps and a number of Turks.

De Carro now realized that Turkey could be used as a transmission point for India. He made two glass plates, one with a shallow concavity, and smeared them with oil. He cut a piece of lint the exact size of the concavity, soaked it in cowpox lymph, covered it with the second plate, sealed the edges, and protected the whole with several layers of wax. De Carro sent the package to Lord Elgin who forwarded it to Baghdad, where it arrived on 31 March 1802. Here a number of people were vaccinated from the lint, the glass plates cleaned, and a fresh supply of lymph packed in a similar manner. The parcel was next sent to Bussora on the Persian Gulf and the process repeated. From Bussora the fresh vaccine travelled on board the ship *Recovery* to Bombay where Dr Helenius Scott received it on 14 June, after a voyage of three weeks. Scott vaccinated twenty people, including his three children, but the lymph had lost potency and only one vaccination 'took'. This case provided enough lymph for a new series and vaccine was successfully sent from Bombay to Madras and Ceylon.

The Indian lymph originated from Berkeley in Gloucestershire. Jenner had taken cowpox matter from one of his first subjects, a girl named Hannah Excell, and sent it in a quill to Henry Cline. Pearson received his supply from Cline and forwarded a sample to de Carro in Vienna. Thus the original 'Jenner strain' travelled to Asia. But a second strain became much more widely distributed. This strain originated at the London Smallpox and Inoculation Hospital and is probably the one most extensively used for the greater part of the nineteenth century. Dr William Woodville found two cows suffering from cowpox at a dairy in Gray's Inn Lane on 20 January 1799. He immediately vaccinated seven subjects at the Smallpox Hospital, and then inoculated all seven with matter from a small-pox pustule, three of them after an interval of only five days. He next vaccinated a first series of 200 from the original seven and later a second series of 300. Most of these 500 people were inoculated with smallpox. Woodville reported 'in several instances, the cowpox has proved a very severe disease. In three or four cases out of five hundred, the patient has been in considerable danger, and one child actually died.'

Jenner was furious. He had purposely delayed test smallpox inocula-tion for over a month in his own trials. He believed that Woodville's vaccine had become contaminated with smallpox virus, either because of the early inoculation or because vaccination had been performed in a smallpox hospital. Jenner must be right. In many instances the resultant disease was smallpox, evidenced by the severity. Woodville distributed his strain widely; by 1836 it had passaged through more than 2,000 removes in England alone. Some was forwarded via the Vaccination Hospital at Bath to Professor Benjamin Waterhouse of Boston, USA, and became disseminated throughout North America. The late Dr A. H. Gale, an authority on infectious disease, pointed out that the modern virus of *Vaccinia* bears more resemblance to the smallpox virus than to that of cowpox. Gale believed 'that the bringing together of cowpox and smallpox virus did in some way produce a modified smallpox virus which by an empirical process of selection on the part of the vaccinators gradually became safer and safer'. Woodville confirms this view in his own words 'if the matter of the cowpox, used for the purpose of inoculation, were only taken from those in whom the disease appeared in a very mild form, the result would be more favourable than in the statement here given'. Woodville muddled Jenner's careful work and must bear much of the blame for the angry vaccination controversy.

The quality of lymph naturally fell under suspicion. In 1807 Parliament ordered the Royal College of Physicians to organize and superintend a central institution for distributing vaccine to every part of the British Dominions. Jenner helped to set up the National Vaccine Establishment and gave advice from time to time. The College surrendered responsibility to the Privy Council in 1861. Ten years later the Local Government Board took over and in 1919 it came under the Ministry of Health.

All vaccinations were performed by the arm-to-arm method until 1881. Continued passage through the human resulted in attenuation and increased risk of transmitting erysipelas, tuberculosis and syphilis. Calf-to-arm, using a purposely infected animal, started at the Government Animal Vaccination Establishment and lymph was sent out on ivory points. It proved very uncertain. In 1891 Dr S. A. Monckton Copeman became a Medical Inspector of the Local Government Board under Sir Richard Thorne Thorne, Principal Medical Officer. Copeman investigated the problem of ensuring viability of the vaccine while destroying extraneous microorganisms. He tried heat and then turned to a method tentatively suggested by Dr R. R. Cheyne in 1850. Cheyne found that glycerine would prolong the life of vaccine. Copeman showed that addition of 50 per cent glycerine in distilled water not only preserved activity but killed the more dangerous extraneous microorganisms. The first distribution of 'glycerinated calf's lymph' began in January 1895, although provision was made for a supply of 'humanized' lymph for those who objected to inoculation with animal matter. Demand for humanized lymph proved small and supply was discontinued in 1899. A Government Lymph Establishment for controlled production and standardization of calf's lymph started work in 1907. The Establishment closed in 1946.

Opposition to vaccination largely centred on the question of compulsion, always a tender subject in a free democracy. The 'animal' objection also played a part. Vaccination tended to be approved by the educated classes while the more conservative lower orders preferred variolation. The majority of doctors declined to inoculate with smallpox, so the practice passed into the hands of unqualified persons. The first attempt to legislate against variolation came in 1808 'whereas the inoculation for the disorder called the smallpox, according to the old or Suttonian method, cannot be practised without the utmost danger of communicating and diffusing the infection . . .'. The Bill, which failed to pass, demanded notification and compulsory isolation of all smallpox cases. The National Vaccination Establishment promoted a similar Bill in 1813. In 1814 came a proposal to make vaccination compulsory among the poor while leaving the richer classes freedom of choice. The epidemic of 1837—40 revived the battle. There were over 16,000 deaths in 1838, 9,000 in 1839 and 10,000 in 1840, the great majority among infants and young children of the working class. Thomas Wakley, MP, editor of the *Lancet*, laid the blame squarely upon variolation, arguing that the epidemic would not have occurred had the practice been prohibited. The Houses accepted Wakley's argument and enacted a law making inoculation of smallpox a felony. The same Act ordered vaccination of children at the ratepayers' expense, but only if parents so desired. In 1853 a new Act made vaccination of infants compulsory, but it had little value because no machinery for enforcement existed.

About half the children born in British towns were vaccinated between 1800 and 1870. In the same period the mortality of smallpox fell from an estimated 3,000—4,000 per million population to 300 per million. The critical period is 1870—3, the most important years in the history of vaccination. We know the genesis of the 1870 epidemic. It was part of a general pandemic which started in 1869. The year of 1870 is the Franco-Prussian War. Compulsory vaccination had been introduced by the more authoritarian states of Europe at an early date, one of the first being Bavaria in 1807. Compulsion became general throughout Germany and army recruits were revaccinated. France did not introduce compulsory vaccination either for the civilian population or the armed forces. During the war 4,835 cases of smallpox with 278 deaths occurred in the German armies. Among French prisoners of war *alone*, smallpox caused 1,963 deaths in 14,178 cases. French refugees brought the infection to England. Introduction from the Continent was inevitable, but this is the first known instance of the appearance of smallpox as an exotic disease in Britain.

The epidemic caused 44,079 deaths in England, nearly a quarter being in London. Epidemiology had by now become a rather more exact science; the outbreak had been anticipated because of an unusually high incidence on the Continent in 1869. Two years previously, an Act had been passed empowering Boards of Guardians to *enforce* infant vaccination. In 1870 the Privy Council warned local authorities to be diligent and a large scale programme resulted. At first sight, the high mortality suggests that vaccination failed, but this is not so. Dr E. C. Seaton reported to the Local Government Board that the average mortality was 148 per 100,000 in London compared with an average 400—500 per 100,000 in the pre-vaccination period. Seaton also drew attention to the eagerness of the population for vaccination in a time of epidemic. In the peak year, 1871, 821,856 children were born in England and Wales. Of these 78,594 died before they could be vaccinated. In all 93.92 per cent of the remainder were successfully treated. This is a quite remarkable record when one remembers that the appointment of Vaccination Officers had not yet become compulsory.

After 1871 the whole country was divided into districts each under the charge of a Public Vaccinator, a general practitioner under contract to vaccinate without fee. A Vaccination Officer had the duty of making the necessary arrangements and of ensuring that all children in his district received treatment. Between 1871 and 1888 about 20 per cent of children escaped and this figure rose to almost 30 per cent in 1897. Partly because so many parents were unwilling and partly because of public antagonism to any form of compulsion, Parliament introduced a 'conscience clause', whereby exemption could be claimed after satisfying two Justices or a Stipendiary Magistrate that vaccination might adversely affect the child's health. The last major smallpox epidemic occurred in 1902—3 when many doctors ascribed the outbreak to the conscience clause. There is little reason to believe in any connection, and the Government did not do so, for exemption was made easier in 1907. A rapid reduction in the number of vaccinations followed, from 63 per cent of children in 1908 to below 50 per cent in 1914 and 34 per cent in 1939. Compulsion ended on 5 July 1948.

No accurate figures for the incidence of smallpox are available until 1899 when compulsory notification was introduced. From 1911 until 1921 annual notifications varied between a high of 315 and a low of 7, deaths varying between 30 and 2. Notifications greatly increased in the next decade 1922—32, with a peak of 14,767 in 1927. But deaths did not parallel notifications: only 47 people died in 1927. On the 1911—21 ratio, the expected deaths would have been in excess of 400. The high incidence and low mortality was attributed to import of mild smallpox or alastrim from America. In April 1928, while the mild form was prevalent, *Variola major* arrived in Liverpool on board S.S. *Tuscania* from India, causing 35 cases with 11 deaths. This small outbreak of the lethal type was easily contained by rigid isolation and vaccination of all contacts. No cases occurred after the end of May. The epidemic of the minor form could not be contained because many people suffered so slight an illness that they did not even call in a doctor. Incidence was therefore much higher than suggested by the registrations. The epidemic did not die out until the end of 1934. No case of endemic smallpox has been reported since 1934; all the small outbreaks have been traced to imports. Smallpox, from being one of the greater killers, has become a rare exotic disease.

Jenner's introduction of vaccination stands out as one of the most beneficial in the history of social medicine. He did not know the cause of disease but his work is the starting point, and is recognized as the starting point, of attempts to combat infection by immunization. In 1880, when he had discovered the existence of pathogenic microorganisms, Louis Pasteur resumed where Jenner had been forced by lack of knowledge to leave off. His successful production of a vaccine against rabies focused attention on the methods by which the body naturally protects itself against infection. From his work there developed not only the protective vaccines but also the antitoxins used successfully in the treatment of developed disease. Diphtheria, for instance, kills by means of toxic products elaborated in the bodies of bacilli and passed into the patient's bloodstream. The toxin can be freed from bacilli by filtration. The filtrate, injected in sub-lethal doses into rabbits, produces a natural body reaction and the serum of the rabbit's blood now contains quantities of a substance capable of neutralizing the diphtheria toxin. Antitoxic serum, first used in 1891, reduced the death rate from diphtheria in London fever hospitals from 63 per cent of cases in 1894 to under 12 per cent in 1910.

Jenner's work and the train of events which he initiated has changed the pattern of infectious disease. He also effected something in the nature of a social revolution. Vaccination induced government action. For the first time in history, the attempt was made to eradicate disease on a national scale.* Individual freedom of choice was sacrificed in the interests of the community. The decision to enforce vaccination is controversial. A historian, Dr Charles Creighton, has denied that vaccination accelerated the end of a disease already starting to decline before the method had been introduced. A medical officer of health, Dr Killick Millard, declared compulsory vaccination of infants, without revaccination at five-year intervals, to be dangerous because it left an inadequately protected population. They might themselves only suffer a mild attack, as may have happened in the 1927 outbreak, but were still capable of producing the severe disease in people who had never been vaccinated. Dr Gale believed that the nineteenth century vaccinators used an attenuated strain of smallpox virus which derived from contamination of *Variola major* with *Variola vaccinae*. These views should command respect, just as should the opposite belief that large scale compulsory vaccination changed smallpox from a common endemic to a rare exotic infection. Not even the widest divergence of opinion upon the merits of vaccination can modify the indisputable fact that compulsory vaccination is the first massive endeavour to vanquish disease. As such, the prevention of smallpox is a landmark in social history.

---

* This statement is perhaps debatable if applied solely to Britain, since Chadwick's sanitary reforms antedate compulsory vaccination. It is not debatable if applied more generally to include Europe.

6   Cholera and sanitary reform

Sir George Newman, Chief Medical Officer of Health, wrote in 1927

Our public health service is the direct offspring of the original Poor
Law service, and sprang out of the fuller appreciation of the close
relationship between the *life* and *occupation* of the poor, and their
disease and early mortality. Such was the ground of their discontent.
But alarm also played its part. For the ravages of cholera in its four
principal invasions of this country in 1831, 1848, 1853 and 1866
had proved a solemn warning to all men that, unless greater
attention was given to sanitation, the country was unsafe.

The middle of the eighteenth century saw the beginning of a great
change in the conditions under which men had lived for more than 1,000
years. World population began to rise quickly, from about 750 million in
1750 to over 900 million in 1800 and 1,200 million in 1850. During this
century, the population of England and Wales rose from 8 million to 18
million. Every year it became necessary to feed and to house an additional
100,000 people. The problem was greater than the figure suggests. As the
Industrial Revolution quickened, there developed a swiftly accelerating
movement from country to town. The villages and market cities of a
farming economy burst their bounds, sprawled over the countryside until,
in many districts, the intervening fields disappeared and individual hamlets
lost identity to become parish names in one coalescent mass.

Britain had managed its sanitary arrangements quite well for a
number of centuries, drawing water from relatively unpolluted sources,
disposing of waste without difficulty. The village drew water from wells
and streams, distributed excreta over the fields. Prolonged drought caused
a shortage of water and a stink. 'Fever', never entirely absent from the
rural community, erupted into local epidemics. Infant mortality would rise
and the medical man talk wisely of 'summer diarrhoea' or 'infantile
cholera'. When the rain came, as it always did, the water level of surface
wells rose quickly, dried ordure leached into the soil, and the village
reverted to its normal British condition of too wet rather than too dry.
The system was based on the natural instinct of higher animals to
defaecate away from their lairs and the rules laid down by Moses for his
Israelites. It had worked for centuries without producing unbearable conditions and persisted in remoter country districts until almost the present

day, until the thatched hovel with its unreliable well and earth privy
became the desirable residence ripe for conversion.

The system even worked in small towns which had invariably grown
up around an abundant water supply and where fields for disposal of waste
lay at the gates. The danger existed that a town might find it more labour-
saving to use its river both as a source of drinking water and a means of
removing excreta. A swiftly flowing stream carried noxious matter away
from the town and the risk of contamination was not high. A tidal river,
such as the Thames at London or the Avon at Bristol, returned a large part
of such noxious matter on the incoming flow and increased the chance of
pollution. When towns started to expand and sprawl across the countryside, difficulty of disposal intensified the risk that waste would enter the
river. Use of steam power in industrial areas diminished an already
inadequate water supply, while the effluent from mills added further
pollution to the source. By 1831 no large manufacturing town in England
possessed water entirely safe to drink and rivers in these areas had become
so polluted that fish could no longer survive.

Some towns supplied piped water under low pressure either to street
conduits or into houses. Larger towns possessed a few sewers, designed
solely to carry off flood water from the roads. Built of brick, with level
floors, flat roofs and straight sides, these 'sewers of deposit' were dry or
almost dry except in times of heavy rain, when the flow of water became
strong enough to carry away accumulations of sludge which entered from
the street drains. In dry weather deposits could be removed only by break-
ing through the roof. The outfall of the sewer was into a river. Sewers
harboured vermin but were fairly safe so long as householders used dry
privies, the contents of which could be removed by hand and carted away.
The water closet, which came into limited use during the last half of the
eighteenth century, added a potent cause of infection. A householder
desiring to instal a water closet must obtain permission from the
Commissioner of Sewers to make a connection, which took the form of a
permeable brick-built drain without traps. Effluent from the water closet
lodged in the rough brickwork and stagnated in the dry sewer, to be
washed at infrequent intervals into the river from which the town drew it
supply of water.

More and more houses had to be built as the country population
moved into the town. The houses must be close to the mill, for neither
master nor worker desired that time should be wasted on travel. A mill
could not start work until houses had been provided for the operatives.
Housing became an urgent problem. Contractors supplied the demand as
quickly as possible. They used available land close to the mill to the best
advantage, cramming a maximum number of dwellings into the restricted
space. Since speed was essential, they did not waste time digging out
foundations, building weight-supporting walls, and erecting tower blocks.
They built skimpily of readily available material, back-to-back in rows or
surrounding narrow yards. The new houses were serviced on the same
principle as the village dwelling, one house or part house to a family with a

shared water supply and outside privies, often no more than a single earth closet to each court or row of houses. Living conditions were no worse, and perhaps a little better, than those to which families had been accustomed in the villages. As time went on, house building could not keep pace with the influx into towns, nor was there any more land available close to the expanding mills, which must necessarily be sited beside a river or canal. Taking in lodgers and sub-letting became the rule. Few families occupied more than a single room, and a two-roomed house might contain as many as twenty people. Cleanliness, privacy, decency, proper sanitation and water supply were all impossible in conditions such as these. The uncleaned privies, in daily use by dozens of people, overflowed and filled the courts with a morass of excrement. This soaked through the ground to contaminate the shallow wells from which the inhabitants drew a scanty supply of water.

Conditions in the industrial slums became disgusting beyond belief. From the sanitary point of view, the wealthy town dweller was not in much better case. He had privacy, space to move, the fine furniture and copious diet that money can buy. Money could not buy exemption from the dangers lying around. His water was no safer than that of the slum. The newly built mansions of Belgravia reeked of drains. Whole streets of middle-class houses contained not a single bath and the water, if piped at all, trickled into the cisterns for two or three hours a day on three days a week. When the scientist Lyon Playfair examined the sanitation of Buckingham Palace he found so many defects that the Government suppressed his report. Typhoid fever attacked not only the poor worker but the highest in the land. It caused the death of Albert the Prince Consort and, ten years later, very nearly killed his son, the future King Edward VII.

We should rid our minds of political indoctrination at this point. Blame for the hideous state of early nineteenth century industrial England must not wholly be laid upon the shoulders of grasping employers and profit-seeking contractors. Slum conditions in the growing towns resulted from two primary errors. The first was the widely held belief that rapid 'progress' is beneficial to a community. The second was the fallacy that a town is only a large-scale village. Hindsight shows us that great damage was caused by the too rapid advance of the Industrial Revolution. Only by calling a halt, making a deliberate pause for constructive planning, could that damage have been avoided. Robert Owen tried to induce government action on these lines in 1817 but failed. There are many who believe that a period of digestion in our own age of rapidly advancing scientific technology might be beneficial. The majority hold that 'progress' cannot be halted. A Tudor autocrat could, and probably would, have accepted Owen's plans and slowed the process by insisting on adequate amenities for the workers before a mill started production. A parliamentary government, mesmerized by the vast increase in national wealth, failed to understand that wealth was bought at the expense of the nation's health. Widespread epidemics provided the spur with which doctors and social reformers drove ministers to action. Legislation quickly followed.

It is a mistake to believe that the agricultural labourer was better off than the industrial worker. All the major evils of the industrial town already existed in the agricultural village. Underfed families lived in overcrowded hovels, women and children worked in the fields, labourers toiled from dawn to dusk at a starvation wage. A child of seven scaring crows on a bleak hillside from first light until nightfall in midwinter does not command the same sympathy as a child of that age labouring in a mill. We remember the overseer's strap but we forget the farmer's whip. We are not so horrified by the picture of a pregnant woman engaged in the backbreaking task of hand-weeding a cornfield as we are by that of her sister harnessed to a coal truck underground. The city-dweller's cloud cuckoo land of a rural Arcady, a Merrie England which never existed, has blinded our eyes to the fact that every evil of the industrial town originated in the agricultural village and depended upon the transfer, not of people only but of their manner of living. This way of life did not become insupportable in the village because communities were small, houses widely separated, and work performed in the open air. The disaster of widespread disease became inevitable when the community was cramped for space, houses lay cheek by jowl, and workers toiled for long hours in an enclosed atmosphere. Late nineteenth century legislation benefited the townsman while leaving the sordid life of the countryman almost unaffected. This is why the town became more healthy than the village at the end of the nineteenth century.

Nor can the blame be ascribed to lack of social conscience. Innumerable gin palaces and a vast consumption of alcohol did much to mislead those who desired betterment of living conditions. They did not appreciate that drink provided the only means of escape. In the absence of clubs or organized sport, in face of overcrowded dwellings and illiteracy, the public house was the only place of relaxation. Philanthropists tended to put all blame on the demon alcohol and argued that workers must be overpaid, and so able to afford better living, if they could waste money on excessive quantities of beer and spirits. The argument contained a grain of truth. The majority of employed families did enjoy an income more than sufficient to provide food and lodging. But there was literally nothing upon which the worker could spend his surplus except alcohol and the fellowship of the pub.

The educated middle class had no knowledge of what was happening in the industrial slums. It is easy to blame them because they did not go to look, just as it is easy to blame the modern package tourist because he prefers sunbathing at his luxury hotel to investigating conditions of life in the back streets of a Portuguese or Spanish town. The nineteenth century citizen believed what he was told. Here we can instance the census returns, which gave the impression that housing kept pace with demand. The respectable householder did not know that every occupancy was counted as a separate dwelling, even though there might be four or more occupancies under one roof. Not until 1842 was the bourgeois class shocked into some understanding by Chadwick's revelations. Then social conscience awoke, but by that time conditions had become so bad that the task of cleaning up the mess occupied many years.

The prevalent ideas of the medical profession upon the cause of disease did not help. During the late eighteenth century doctors noticed that 'fever' was more common in the slums than in upper-class districts. They evolved the pythogenic theory, or theory of miasma, which held all disease to be due to bad air. Many of them discarded the old concept of contagion, a direct spread from person to person. The pythogenic theory, if put into stringent practice, might have exerted a beneficial effect by insisting upon a better standard of cleanliness. But any measures taken would have been directed more against fouling of the air and less against the real evils of contaminated water supply and bad sanitation. When the relation between disease and infected water had been clearly shown, legislation to ensure a clean supply soon followed.

The first national Board of Health, instituted by Government to minimize risk of disease entering Britain, dates from 1804 when yellow fever threatened to invade. Nations have tried to prevent import of exotic diseases from quite early times. In 1374 the Venetian republic ordered inspection and exclusion of infected ships. Three years later the town of Ragusa, Sicily, required persons suspected to be suffering from disease to be detained for thirty days before entering the gates. The port authorities of Marseilles extended the period to forty days in 1383 and, in 1403, Venice enacted that travellers from the Levant must be isolated in a detention hospital for the same period, *quaranta giorni*, from which the word quarantine is derived. The first quarantine regulations for ships entering British ports date from 1742. A severe epidemic of yellow fever at Gibraltar in the early years of the nineteenth century aroused apprehension that the dreaded disease might enter British ports. In December 1804 the Privy Council desired the Royal College of Physicians to suggest measures to limit or prevent the catastrophe. The physicians advised a strict quarantine of shipping and the establishment of a Board of Health empowered to make regulations. The Board started work in May 1805 as a committee of the Privy Council. It made preventive rules, set up a Centre of Epidemic Intelligence for gathering information from all parts of the world, and took over several buildings as isolation hospitals. Reports collected from Epidemic Intelligence Officers threw new light on the epidemiology of yellow fever and helped to reduce mortality on the West Indian station where the death toll had been almost 50 per cent among new recruits. The threat of yellow fever in Britain did not materialize and the Board was dissolved on 8 August 1806. It set the pattern for future Boards and is the first parent of our Ministry of Health and Social Security.

Cholera, an Asiatic disease, has never been endemic in Britain. Some authorities hold that introductions of cholera may have caused European epidemics at a quite early date. It is difficult to understand why these should have aroused so little comment nor, in view of the later story, is it easy to believe that transmission from the East could occur until communications became rapid. The history is not clear, even in India. The first recognizable description dates from around 400 BC. An expedition led by Vasco da Gama in 1498 suffered from a virulent illness after arriving in India and this is thought to have been cholera, although there is no good evidence as to its nature. The infection was certainly prevalent in Madras during the years 1770—90. In June 1814 it appeared among native troops on a march of many hundreds of miles from Trichinopoly, a district of Madras, to Jaunpur or Jawalpur, both towns in the United Provinces, the latter standing on the River Ganges. In 1817 cholera broke out with great violence over the whole Ganges delta, which became notorious as a focus. Medical men in the area stated that it had not been seen in the delta before 1817 and considered it a new disease. A possible explanation is that cholera was endemic in Central India, then largely unexplored by the European, and made its way down river to the coast, to be disseminated by troop movements and coastal shipping.

Cholera was on the move at the beginning of the nineteenth century. In 1817—18 came the first known export from India, eastward to China and the Philippines, south to Mauritius and Reunion, north-west to Persia and Turkey. By 1826 a pandemic covered the whole of China, Japan and Asiatic Russia. Poland, Germany, Austria and Sweden were all infected in 1829. The first English cases appeared at Sunderland in October 1831 and the whole of Europe and the British Isles had been invaded by the winter of 1832—3. Quebec and New York received cholera by ship in 1832 and the disease spread slowly south to Mexico. Thus thirteen years elapsed between export from India and invasion of Britain. Here is a pattern quite different from that of bubonic plague, which travelled the length of Europe in less than a year. The general progress of cholera was slow and it travelled far more quickly by ship than by overland routes. We cannot improve upon the account written by John Snow in 1849:

> There are certain circumstances, however, connected with the progress of cholera, which may be stated in a general way. It travels along the great tracks of human intercourse, never going faster than people travel, and generally much more slowly. In extending to a fresh island or continent, it always appears first at a seaport. It never attacks the crews of ships going from a country free from cholera to one where the disease is prevailing, till they have entered a port, or had intercourse with the shore. Its exact progress from town to town cannot always be traced; but it has never appeared except where there has been ample opportunity for it to be conveyed by human intercourse.

This insidious progress, moving across Europe at the rate of about eight kilometres (five miles) a day, gave the British authorities time to initiate action. They had the pattern of the 1805 Board of Health, although it had never functioned during a developed epidemic. The Board must work through existing local organizations. The only ones available were composed of parish officers and justices of the peace, whose primary duty was to implement the provisions of the Poor Law under the titular control of the Privy Council. The system dated from the reign of Elizabeth

I and, during the course of years, had become so decentralized that every parish was virtually a self-governing unit.

In January 1831 Charles Greville, Clerk of the Privy Council, asked Dr Walker of St Petersburg for a description of the epidemic in that city. Walker replied in March with a second-hand account. Cholera reached the Baltic coast in early summer and on 17 June Greville sent Dr William Russell and Dr David Barry to investigate and make a report. Four days later, on 21 June, a Central Board of Health was established under the Privy Council. The authorities made a serious mistake in appointing leading members of the medical profession and high officials to the Board, instead of waiting for the return of Barry and Russell or finding Indian doctors who had some experience. The Board met under the presidency of Sir Henry Halford, who is only memorable as the last bearer of the Gold Headed Cane, a symbol of office in the Royal College of Physicians. However, the Board worked hard, meeting almost daily from 21 June until 11 November 1831. They were required to prepare 'such Rules and Regulations as they may deem most effectual for the adoption of the most approved method of guarding against the cholera'. Their task might have been simpler and more useful had any member seen a case of cholera or had knowledge of the cause. They were not deterred. By 29 June the Board had prepared recommendations and forwarded them to the Privy Council. This historic document is the first attempt to influence public health through local government.

> As there are strong reasons for believing that the disease called *Cholera Morbus* now prevailing in Russia and the North of Europe is infectious, it is of the utmost importance that the very first cases that appear should be known as early as possible and that concealment of the sick should be guarded against. With this view it is submitted that in every Town or Village commencing with those on the Coast there should be established a local Board of Health to consist of the Chief Magistrate and Clergymen, one or more of the Professional Gentlemen and Principal Inhabitants. One of the medical members to be appointed to correspond with the Board of Health in London. Every Town under such circumstances should be immediately divided into Districts, having a District committee of two or three members, one of them of the Medical Profession, to watch over its health and to give the earliest information to the Board of Health of the Town whose instructions they will carry into effect.
>
> In each Town or its Neighbourhood one or more places to be immediately pointed out as places to which every case of the disease as soon as detected might be removed in conveyances appropriated exclusively for the purpose. For the higher classes who can pay for other accommodation, houses to be hired in airy and detached Situations under the Control of the Magistrates.
>
> The Houses from which the Sick Persons have been removed should be purified in the following manner. The wearing apparel and household furniture should be thoroughly washed and scoured, the walls

and ceilings limewashed, the doors and windows of each apartment left open for many days.

The Occupiers of each House where the Disease may occur or be supposed to have occurred to report to the District Committee of Health in order that the Professional Member may immediately visit, report, and if necessary cause the patient to be removed to the place allotted for the sick. The names and residences of each of the Members of the District Committee of Health to be fixed on the doors of the Church or other conspicuous place.

Further and more detailed instructions and likewise descriptions of the disease called *Cholera Morbus* will be transmitted hereafter.

Further recommendations of the Board included the appointment of officers known as 'expurgators' with the duty of removing sufferers to lazarettos and contacts to isolation hospitals. The Board pointed out that police and military must be available to prevent attacks upon the expurgators or attempts at rescue of patients. They suggested imposition of fines for concealment and rewards for detection. The Privy Council, now thoroughly alarmed by their child's aggressiveness, deliberated for a month before permitting the Board to circulate such part of their regulations as they thought necessary 'provided they are not contrary to law', at the same time emphasizing that they had no power to implement the regulations until cholera had arrived in the country. On 3 September Sir Henry Halford outlined the Board's proposals in the *Lancet*, omitting mention of expurgators or fines. Thomas Wakley, the radical editor, launched a violent attack upon the whole scheme and its originators.

Despite opposition from medical practitioners and misgivings of the Privy Council, towns and rural districts now began to set up local Boards of Health in anticipation. They were not altogether an innovation. Manchester had possessed an unofficial Board since 1794 and Newcastle formed one in June 1831, before the Privy Council proposals had been published. On 12 October danger became acute with the appearance of cholera at Hamburg, a port of regular communication with the British Isles. The Privy Council met on the morning of 20 October to consider putting the rules into operation. An unknown but intelligent Privy Councillor then pointed out that, although the physicians had urged a close watch on coastal towns and immediate isolation of suspects, they had omitted to give any indication of how a case of cholera was to be recognized. The Board, then in session, received an urgent letter at 4.30 pm but found it necessary to adjourn and seek the required information. They met again at 10.30 pm and embodied their findings in a document which was immediately despatched from the Board's meeting place at the Royal College of Physicians in Pall Mall to the Privy Council Office in Whitehall. From Whitehall the Rules and regulations, with an additional statement on the nature and treatment of cholera, was sent to the printers in time to appear in the *London Gazette* of the same date, 20 October.

A week later, 27 October, James Kell, an army surgeon, reported the first British death from cholera at Sunderland. Four more deaths were reported before 1 November. The Home Secretary, Lord Melbourne, issued instructions to magistrates that the regulations as promulgated on 20 October must now be enforced. Local Boards had been set up in more than twenty-five towns by 14 November. The Privy Council decided that a Central Board containing members who knew something of cholera might be useful, and dismissed the physicians on the pretext that they were too busy to spare the time for the almost permanent session now required. The new Board contained Drs Russell and Barry, Edward Stewart a full-time customs official, and Sir William Pym of the quarantine service. The Board was full-time and did not confine itself to meetings in Whitehall. Barry left immediately for Sunderland and other members travelled about the country encouraging formation of Local Boards, instituting isolation hospitals, and advising on segregation and treatment. By February 1832 the Central Board employed four deputy inspectors-general of hospitals, twenty-one medical officers and seventeen surgeons. At the end of the epidemic these officers were advising over 1,200 local Boards of Health, of which 822 were in England and Wales and some 400 in Scotland. The epidemic caused about 22,000 deaths before the beginning of June 1832. Then mortality started to decline and virtually ended in December, when the Central Board of Health was dissolved. In February 1832 the Cholera Prevention Act permitted direction by Orders in Council. Among other directives are: provision of nurses and medicines to the sick poor in their own homes; dispensaries; cleansing of infected houses; removal of offal and filth; covering over drains and cesspools; abatement of nuisances in general; burial of persons who died of cholera outside parish boundaries; destruction of clothing, bedding, and other articles belonging to the deceased. This wise legislation broke down in practice because local authorities, although empowered to take action, did not possess the physical means of enforcement. Further, all payments had to be made from parish rates, which were already overburdened by outdoor relief.

In 1795 Berkshire magistrates, meeting at Speenhamland, had tied agricultural wages to the cost of bread and decreed that any further money required by a worker must be levied on the parish. This unwise decision subsidized farmers, pauperized labourers, and diverted rates from their legal purpose of supporting the poor. The 1831–2 epidemic left apprehension that slum areas, whether in country or town, formed a breeding ground of disease and social unrest. Fear was intensified by the riots preceding the 1832 Reform Act and the Government set up a Royal Commission to enquire into the working of the Poor Law, the primary purpose being to find a cheaper system of relief. The most able and industrious member of the Commission, Nassau Senior, invited the help of Edwin Chadwick, a lawyer-journalist who had acted as Jeremy Bentham's secretary.

Chadwick outlined a scheme to limit outdoor relief and prevent farmers employing cheap labour at the public expense. He proposed to cut relief to subsistence level and combine it with an irksome discipline, thus deterring the able-bodied worker who could fend for himself. The whole parish rate might then be available for such as were unable to work, the sick, the young, the aged, and the real unemployed. He hoped that these measures would result in a large migration of agricultural labourers from the highly pauperized south to the industrial north where labour was in demand and wages higher. Chadwick advised a series of specialized hospitals for care of the necessitous classes, asylums for the aged and impotent, orphanages for children, workhouses for able-bodied persons unable to find work. As measures tending to prevent pauperism, he advocated free elementary education and sanitary regulations of the kind laid down by the obsolescent Central Board of Health. He also devised the mechanism necessary to implement his proposals, a central Poor Law Commission of three members employing a body of paid itinerant inspectors and local overseers. The old inefficient system by which each parish managed its own poor law affairs would cease, to be replaced by a compulsory amalgamation of parishes into a Union with a central workhouse, asylum and orphanage.

The politicians bungled Chadwick's scheme by their impatience. They adopted his repressive measures but omitted mention of free education and sanitation. They sanctioned his Commission of three members, but refused paid inspectors and overseers, leaving management of the Union to local representatives elected by the ratepayers. Few, if any, authorities provided separate institutions as Chadwick had envisaged. Old, young, sick and able-bodied, rigidly segregated by sex, inadequately fed, bullied by tyrannical Masters and Matrons, were herded together into a single building, the Union of hated memory.

Chadwick now became Secretary of the new Poor Law Commission and used his office as a means of gathering information. In 1836 when the Registration of Death Bill came before Parliament, he secured introduction of a clause requiring registrars to insert the *cause* of death. When the Bill became law, he persuaded the first Registrar General, T. H. Lister, to appoint a statistician, William Farr. In 1838, the first full year of registration, there occurred a major epidemic of typhus fever. About 14,000 people fell sick in London alone, of whom 1,281 died. Some Union authorities noted a relation between the incidence of fever and the level of poor-rate. In a few instances they took advantage of the Cholera Prevention Act and indicted landlords who refused to abate nuisances. The cost of prosecution was charged to the poor-rate, but auditors refused to allow this as a reasonable expense. The dispute was naturally taken to the Secretary of the Poor Law Commission. Chadwick saw the chance for an investigation, with the possible outcome of introducing the sanitary reforms omitted from his first scheme.

He enlisted the help of three doctors, Neill Arnott, James Kay (later Kay-Shuttleworth) and Thomas Southwood Smith. They examined conditions obtaining in the worst fever districts and concluded that high incidence was largely caused by dirty habits and drunkenness, but that the poor could do little to better themselves while living conditions remained filthy. The doctors recommended that powers be given to Poor Law Guardians to cleanse stagnant pools and ditches, inspect lodging houses, and prosecute any person failing to abate nuisances. In'August 1839 the Bishop of London moved in the House of Lords for an extended enquiry. This was largely undertaken by Chadwick himself between 1839 and 1842.

He demanded from Unions not only the number of deaths but the number of cases of infectious (zymotic) disease. In all, he examined returns from 553 districts. Chadwick prepared 'sanitary maps' which clearly showed both death and disease incidence to be highest in the most overcrowded areas. He took the mortality in eight different places and showed the average age of death to be related to class: forty-three years for gentry, thirty for tradesmen, and twenty-two for labourers. The last, and very low, expectation of life was reflected in the number of widows and orphans receiving relief. In 1840 the figures were 112,000 orphans and 43,000 widows. He estimated that 100,000 had been orphaned and 27,000 widowed through death of the bread-winner from zymotic disease. Chadwick concluded that disease was propagated among the labouring class by atmospheric pollution, resulting from filth, overcrowding, lack of drainage, and defective water supply. He warned that overcrowding produced the evils of bastardy and incest and forced children onto the streets where they soon learned to thieve, beg, and sell themselves as prostitutes. He pointed the danger of a short life expectancy among labourers. Disease thinned the ranks of higher age groups, leaving a young, passionate and dangerous population, easily deceived by anarchist fallacies. Here lay the reason why Chartism, born in the slums, emerged to threaten the established order. Chadwick's biographer, R. A. Lewis, remarks that he 'drew his respectable hearers to the edge of the pit and bade them observe the monsters they were breeding beneath their feet'.

Published under the title *Report of an Inquiry into the Sanitary Conditions of the Labouring Population of Great Britain* on 9 July 1842, the findings of Chadwick and his fellow Commissioners shook Government and bourgeoisie out of their complacency. Implementation of the Report would require legislation and heavy expenditure. The question was referred to a committee, usually known as the Health of Towns Commission, under the chairmanship of the Duke of Buccleuch. Members of the public took independent action. On 11 December 1844 a meeting at Exeter Hall, London, chaired by the Marquess of Normanby, founded the Metropolitan Health of Towns Association. A number of larger cities, among them Liverpool, followed suit. After startling reports by the Commission in 1844 and 1845, several towns introduced private Bills designed to promote better government in their areas. Of these, the Liverpool Sanitary Act, 1846, proved a model for future legislation. The Act not only empowered the Town Council to effect sanitary improvements but created machinery by authorizing appointment of a Medical Officer of Health, a Borough Engineer, and an Inspector of Nuisances. On 1 January 1847 Liverpool appointed Dr William Henry Duncan to be the first Medical Officer of Health in Britain.

Chadwick turned from broad policy to detail. He had no practical knowledge of sanitary engineering and set himself to learn the first principles. He found two efficient advisers in Thomas Hawksley of Nottingham, designer of the Trent River Water Works, and John Roe, a surveyor to the Holborn Sewers Commission. Piped water supply was coming increasingly into use, but the companies were obsessed by the ancient main, a bored elm trunk which split under pressure. For this reason they still supplied water at much the same pressure as in the days of the wooden conduit, although they now used metal piping. Poorer areas were usually provided with a few standpipes but, because of the low mains pressure, they were available for only an hour or two on stated days. Hawksley proved that pressure could be maintained by using iron pipe and that it was economic to provide a constant and unlimited supply of water to working class tenants at a rate of.1*d.* per week.

Next came the problem of sewage disposal. Roe had shown that the old fashioned 'sewer of deposit' could be economically replaced by narrow-bore, self-cleaning drains. This type of sewer, circular or oval in section and running in smooth curves, required a constant flow of water for efficient cleansing and to prevent blockage. This indicated installation of water closets in place of earth privies. But there were two objections. Water closet effluent could not be led by the sewer into rivers without risk of gross contamination. Further, diversion of all sewage into the rivers would result in a large loss of valuable manure.

Chadwick concluded that water supply and sewage disposal depended upon each other. He devised the 'arterio-venous' system, an exchange of country water for town sewage. The system depended upon land-drainage, which had so increased farm production during the last century. Chadwick proposed to pump excess water from agricultural areas into towns, and to fertilize the countryside with liquid town sewage pumped through return pipes. The term 'sewage farm' commemorates his scheme. Water closets now became not only possible but desirable, since the self-cleansing sewer depended upon an adequate flow. Chadwick worked out the economics. A cesspool cost £5 and, in towns, £1 a year for emptying, or roughly 4*d.* a week. For a capital expenditure of £4, a house could be fitted with water closet, sink, water pipe and drain. Translated into terms of rent, these amenities together with a constant and unlimited water supply, could be provided for an additional 2½*d.* a week. Chadwick now turned to administration. He had little trust in elected local authorities or Boards of Guardians. He did not wish to be hampered by a democratic Parliament. Chadwick argued that central control produced more efficient action at the periphery. He visualized implementation of his proposals by local *ad hoc* committees, composed of members nominated by the Crown, and directed by a Central Board responsible only to the Privy Council. The chief executives would be Medical Officers of Health, full-time salaried officials for whom Chadwick prepared a detailed list of rules and duties.

Two things now happened. In 1845 a new epidemic of cholera

started in Kabul and spread west. By 1847 the British government had become seriously alarmed. Second, Chadwick quarrelled with the Poor Law Commissioners and was dismissed from the secretaryship on 8 July 1847. The Prime Minister, Lord John Russell, immediately put him in charge of a special enquiry into the sanitary defects of London, thought to be at particular risk from cholera. His findings added to the government's alarm. Chadwick's proposals had been embodied in a Bill presented to Parliament on 30 March 1847. The Bill failed to pass, was redrafted, and became law under the title of the Public Health Act ('The Chadwick Act') on 31 August 1848. There is no doubt that the threat of cholera, coupled with Chadwick's adverse report on the state of London, led to ill-considered and panic legislation.

The Act greatly extended the power of local authorities and added to their commitments. They became responsible for paving streets and constructing drains and sewers. They were vested with property in all dust, ashes and street refuse, which implied a duty to collect and a right to sell. They had power to buy out any millowner or other person whose buildings formed a barrier to free drainage or ventilation. Local authorities had the duty to procure a supply of water ample for domestic use, cleansing streets, scouring sewers and extinguishing fires. Water might be obtained from private companies or, with the Crown's approval, by purchase. Capital for improvements would be raised by loans on security of the rates. An additional annual rate would be chargeable to occupiers of 'improved' premises.

Existing local authorities were incompetent to carry out these excellent ideas. The Act instituted a General Board of Health, empowered to sanction Local Boards *but only on petition of the ratepayers*. 'Any city, town, borough, parish or place having a known or defined boundary' might be granted a provisional order by the General Board if 'not less than one tenth of the inhabitants rated to the relief of the poor' signed the petition. Only in the worst areas, where the number of deaths annually exceeded an average of twenty-three per thousand of the population, would a Local Board be granted by an Order in Council on the recommendation of the General Board. The General Board had no real power and its administrative status was ill-defined. Chadwick's demand that it be responsible solely to the Privy Council had been refused. Set up by Act of Parliament, the Board formed no part of any ministry and had no spokesman. It had indefinite duties, was responsible to no man, and could count on no support except the goodwill that might or might not be engendered. The General Board consisted of three members, Lord Morpeth, Lord Ashley (later Lord Shaftesbury) and Mr Edwin Chadwick who received a salary. In October 1848 he was joined by his former associate Dr T. Southwood Smith as medical adviser. They held their first meeting on 21 November.

By this time cholera had appeared in Edinburgh, infecting London in December and spreading over the rest of the country before June 1849. The epidemic was worse than in 1831−2. At least 50,000 and probably more nearly 70,000 died in England and Wales. London suffered about 30,000 cases with over 14,000 deaths. Cholera gave to the General Board of Health the authority denied by Parliament. Within three days of their first meeting, sixty-two towns petitioned for application of the Public Health Act. Many more towns asked for inspectors to be sent to adjudicate on nuisances. The Board, inundated with demands for advice, found difficulty in coping. They secured passage of a Nuisances Removal and Diseases Prevention Act, which gave some powers of compulsion in relation to local authorities. The Act could only be enforced in times of emergency such as a cholera epidemic. The General Board was now enabled to order abatement of nuisances, cleansing of streets, disinfecting of houses and to provide isolation hospitals. Chadwick used the Act to recruit a special corps of health visitors, to increase the number of Poor Law surgeons, and to press the advantages of Medical Officers of Health upon local authorities.

The major legacy of the General Board is the Medical Officer of Health. We have already noted that Liverpool appointed the first under a Private Act in January 1847. The City of London adopted the same procedure in the following year when John Simon became Medical Officer. Neither of these posts was full-time; Simon actually combined his duties with an assistant surgeoncy at King's College Hospital and a lectureship in pathology at St Thomas'. This was against Chadwick's advice. In 1848 he persuaded Liverpool, which suffered not only from cholera but also from continual epidemics of typhus because of immigration from famine-stricken Ireland, to make Dr Duncan's appointment into a full-time post at a salary of £750 a year. This was exceptional; there is no other instance of a full-time appointment during the life of the General Board. Local authorities paid very low salaries ranging from £100 to as little as £15 a year. They often made temporary appointments during times of epidemic, paid at a daily rate. The medical profession suspected employment by local authorities, who had shown themselves indifferent as to whether a practitioner did or did not possess a qualification. Even the 1848 Public Health Act laid down that a Medical Officer of Health must be 'a legally qualified medical practitioner *or member of the medical profession*' (author's italics). The latter proviso theoretically permitted quacks or imposters practising as doctors to be legally appointed. As all appointments had to be approved by the General Board, the risk was small but an aura of suspicion remained.

The number of Medical Officers of Health appointed during the life of the General Board 1848—54 is small; only thirty-five towns are known to have petitioned the Board on this head compared with 320 which applied for sanction of Local Boards. The first to appoint under the Act was Leicester (Dr John Buck) in August 1849. Nearly half the thirty-five date from the last four months of 1853, when the third of the great cholera epidemics created panic. The Medical Officers worked under rules laid down by the General Board in a letter signed by Lord Ashley, Edwin Chadwick and T. Southwood Smith. Duties included house-to-house visiting in search of infectious disease, removal of sick from overcrowded tenements, vaccination of smallpox contacts, enquiries into outbreaks of infection in schools and factories, establishing evidence on nuisances, inspection of sanitary improvement works, determining the cause of unexpected death, attendance at all meetings of the Local Board of Health, keeping a diary of all visits and a record of applications, furnishing quarterly and annual reports—quite a lot to expect from a part-time doctor in return for between £15 and £100 a year. The MOH sent his annual reports to the General Board; they provided an excellent overall picture of the state of towns and the kind of improvements made by local authorities.

The General Board of Health did good work but became increasingly unpopular. Chadwick antagonized both medical profession and local authorities by his dictatorial attitude. Public attack mounted at the time when its first period of office, fixed by the Public Health Act at five years, was ending. The 1853—4 cholera epidemic was now in progress and the Government wisely decided, in face of much opposition, to continue the Board's life for another year. On 31 July 1854 a motion to implement the Act for another term was defeated by seventy-four votes to sixty-five. The debate took the form of a venomous attack on Chadwick. One member declared that England wanted to be clean but not to be cleaned by Mr Chadwick. Sir Benjamin Hall said he had been removed from the Poor Law Board for his 'rules of atrocious stringency'. He had 'concocted a pamphlet on sanitary subjects' by means of which he had manoeuvred himself into a position of absolute power on the Board. Hall announced himself to be 'quite at a loss to know what services this man had rendered to the community'. A *Times* leader approving Chadwick's dismissal contained the words 'we prefer to take our chance of cholera and the rest than to be bullied into health'.

There is little doubt that Chadwick's downfall can be, at least partially, attributed to the Board's failure to arrest cholera. Sewage disposal and unlimited water supply will not be regarded as vital necessities if the blame for a fearful epidemic is laid solely upon bad air. There is no evidence that any member of the Board deviated from the common theory of miasma. Yet a pamphlet suggesting the true means by which cholera spreads had been published in 1849. *On the Mode of Communication of Cholera* is by Dr John Snow, a London physician sometimes better remembered as the first specialist anaesthetist.

Early in 1832 Snow, then a nineteen-year old apprentice at Newcastle-on-Tyne, helped during an explosive outbreak of cholera at Killingworth colliery. He decided that neither direct contagion nor bad air transmitted the infection, but that diarrhoea and vomiting, unwashed hands and shared food played a major part. He followed up his idea during the epidemic of 1849 when 140 deaths occurred among 1,000 children at an orphan asylum in Tooting. The children slept two or three in a bed. Snow thought that unaffected children's hands became fouled by excretions and they acquired cholera by sucking their fingers. He suggested that the same mechanism applied to the poor. Whole families had to cook and take meals in the room where a patient lay sick. The profuse cholera evacuations wetted bed linen and the hands of a person attending the victim must become soiled. If that person prepared food, a minute amount of excreta would be ingested by anyone who ate it, thus spreading the disease. Doctors attending patients escaped because they did not eat food in the houses.

Such might be the reason for rapid spread of cholera among the poor, but Snow still had to find a means by which it reached the houses of the rich. He now postulated that cholera evacuations might become mixed 'with the water used for drinking or culinary purposes, either by permeating the ground and getting into wells, or by running along channels and sewers into the rivers from which entire towns are sometimes supplied with water'. The dramatic incident of the Broad Street pump showed Snow that he was on the right track. In 1849 the majority of houses around Golden Square in London were not served with piped water but depended upon 'pump wells', of which that in Broad Street yielded an unusually drinkable supply. At the end of August cholera struck the district, causing over 600 deaths. The outbreak took an explosive form in the Broad Street area, 344 deaths occurring in the four days 1—4 September. Snow investigated eighty-nine deaths in Broad Street and found that all except ten of the dead lived close to the pump and drew their water from the well. Of the remaining ten, five would have been expected to draw water from a nearer source but preferred the Broad Street supply. Three more were children who attended a school served by the pump. There is a curious incident connected with this story which seems to have gone unremarked. Snow records that John Gould, the famous ornithologist, lived near the pump in Broad Street. He returned home from a holiday on Saturday, 2 September, and immediately sent for some water. To his surprise he found that it smelt offensively although perfectly clear and fresh from the well. He did not drink it, nor did his assistant Mr Prince. Gould's servant drank some and was seized with cholera but recovered.

Snow, now fairly sure of his facts, traced the pipelines of various water companies and showed that cholera abounded in districts served by one company but was almost absent in those served by another. In some streets, the pipelines ran side by side, each company serving houses in the same street. Cholera was rife in those served by Company A and infrequent in those served by Company B. An outbreak of cholera occurred in the houses on one side of a road but not upon the other. Water came to the whole street from the innocent Company B. Snow discovered that the first case happened in a house served by a cesspit; this had overflowed and the effluent had seeped into a cracked earthenware main which supplied water to the houses upon that side of the street.

John Snow had proved that cholera is a water-borne disease in 1849. He confirmed his findings during the epidemic of 1853—4. Comparing two of the largest suppliers, he found that the Southwark and Vauxhall Water

Company supplied 40,046 houses in which 1,263 people died from cholera in the seven weeks ending 26 August 1854. This represented a rate of 315 deaths per 10,000 houses. The Lambeth Water Company supplied 26,107 houses in which there were 98 deaths, a rate of 57 per 10,000, less than one-fifth that of the Southwark and Vauxhall. Snow advanced the theory that the *materies morbi* of cholera is a living organism capable of reproduction. Dr William Budd of Bristol came to the same conclusion. In 1849 he investigated the cholera epidemic in Bristol and formed the opinion that the causal agent multiplied in the human intestine and was disseminated by contaminated drinking water. Before working in Bristol, Budd practised in North Tawton, Devon, where a number of cottages had become notorious for the prevalence of 'fever'. Budd not only differentiated 'fever' into typhus fever and typhoid, but showed that the high incidence of the latter was related to a contaminated well serving the cottages. He treated the excreta of typhoid victims with chloride of lime and reduced the incidence. John Snow and William Budd not only proved Chadwick's contention that pure water supply and efficient disposal of sewage is essential to health, but came close to anticipating Pasteur's Germ Theory.

After the dismissal of Lord Shaftesbury, Chadwick and Southwood Smith, the first General Board of Health was reconstituted on a year-to-year tenure with Sir Benjamin Hall as president. Hall appointed an Advisory Medical Council which included the statistician William Farr and the Medical Officer of Health for London John Simon. Working on statistics for the 1849 and 1853 epidemics, compiled by Farr, they determined to prove whether the water-borne theory of Snow and Budd was correct or not. They selected nine London parishes, ranging in social status from affluent to poverty-stricken. The two water companies investigated by Snow supplied and competed in each parish, their mains running side by side in the same streets. The total population had been 466,000 in 1849 and increased to 511,000 in 1854. Investigation showed that in 1853, the two companies supplied 64,580 houses containing 435,077 people. In the 24,854 houses supplied by Lambeth there occurred 611 deaths among 166,906 people, a rate of 37 per 10,000. In the 39,726 houses supplied by the Southwark Company there occurred 3,476 deaths among 268,171 people a rate of 130 per 10,000. This startling confirmation of Snow's figures became even more significant if the Lambeth figure for 1853 was compared to that for 1849, when the Lambeth water was responsible for the death of 1,925 people in a smaller population—three times the mortality in 1853—4. Between the two epidemics Lambeth had adopted the method of sand filtration, introduced by James Simpson, engineer of the Chelsea Water Works, in 1829. The investigators said of the water supplied by Lambeth and by Southwark in 1854 'the former furnishing as good a water as any distributed in London, while the latter was purveying perhaps the filthiest stuff ever drunk by a civilized community'.

John Simon presented the Committee's findings to the General

Board of Health in May 1856. The Board came to an end in 1858. The Public Health Acts of 1858 and 1859 transferred responsibility for health to the Privy Council. The Acts empowered the Privy Council to appoint a Medical Officer with the duty of investigating health problems and preparing reports for presentation to Parliament. John Simon became the first Medical Officer of the Privy Council and remained in office until 1876, five years after public health passed into the care of the Local Government Board. The years of Privy Council control 1858—71 form a period of peace between the General Board's tenure and renewed warfare under the Local Government Board. Chadwick had left behind him a philosophy of public health and the beginnings of an authority to put this philosophy into operation. Snow and others had shown Chadwick to be entirely justified in his struggle for proper sanitation and clean water supply. The Medical Officer of the Privy Council no longer needed to force his recommendations upon unwilling local authorities. He could regard public health as an academic science, making his recommendations directly to Parliament upon whom the responsibility for action devolved. This might have been a time of stagnation. That it blossomed into one of the most fruitful periods in the history of social medicine is due to the genius of John Simon.

Simon possessed in a very marked degree the ability to choose men and to head them as a team. He had no permanent assistant staff; the Privy Council allowed him to appoint inspectors for specific duties, usually at the rate of £3 a day, occasionally on a full-time basis at £800 a year. The majority of the sixteen doctors associated with Simon were young and inexperienced. Almost without exception they rose to high rank in their profession. No less than eight became Fellows of the Royal Society. Only three failed to attain distinction and two of these were sick men.

Members of the team investigated the causes of high mortality. They concluded that an excessive death rate depended upon two causes, tainting of the atmosphere by the products of decomposition and the drinking of impure water. But, although this instigated a drive for proper sanitation and water supply, the investigators soon found these measures were not enough. In 1860—1 research into the occurrence of lung diseases showed that many trades placed workers at risk. From here the team passed to industrial hazards in general, showed small cottage industries to be often as prejudicial to health as employment in the great factories, and issued a report in 1863 *Hurtful or Hurtfully Conducted Occupations*. At the same time two members, Edward Smith and H. J. Hunter, made surveys of diet and housing. Smith showed that the majority of workers suffered from malnutrition, the result of bad domestic education rather than of low purchasing power. Malnutrition combined with poor working and housing conditions to produce national ill-health. Hunter uncovered the worst evils of overcrowding, especially pernicious in the coal-mining areas of the Midlands and North. He found over 300 *single room* occupancies in which the family took in lodgers.

The team next concentrated on the appalling problem of infant mortality which then stood at a national average of about 150 per 1,000 live births. The rate was higher in the working class and very high when the mothers were employed. The investigators discovered the frightful truth that excessive mortality was caused by drugging. Godfrey's Cordial, an opium mixture, was the narcotic in most common use. Sales in Coventry amounted to about ten gallons weekly, enough for 12,000 doses, administered to not more than 3,000 children under two years old. Hunter mapped out five areas where infant mortality ranged between 200 and 260 per 1,000. In all, he found evidence of drugging. In one Fen district of East Anglia, doctors had attributed the high infant death rate to malaria. He found the cause to be the exact opposite, that drainage and tilling had abolished malaria but had created field work for mothers. He met gangs of strapping, well-fed young women coming back from the fields in the evening, having left their babies at home all day. One-third of all illegitimate children died in the first year of life, and one-quarter of all legitimate. Sheer starvation and drugging with opium were the two most common causes. One retail druggist admitted dispensing over 200 lb. of opium a year in the form of pills, penny sticks and Godfrey's Cordial

This work by Simon's inspectors could not have been done without the railways, now covering Britain with a network from city to city. These inspectors travelled everywhere, trying to visit every town, every street and even every house. They gathered information about all serious epidemics, smallpox, diphtheria, typhus fever. They incorporated this mass of information into annual reports upon the state of the national health. By 1866 Simon had gathered an immense body of evidence and the time had come for legislation. He showed himself a skilled diplomat, lobbying Members of Parliament, feeding his own ideas into their minds, flattering them into the self-delusion that they had themselves conceived his plans. Simon's reports initiated the Factory Act and the Workshop Act of 1867, the Sanitary Act, 1866, the Vaccination Act of 1871 and the Artizans and Labourers Dwellings Act ('The Torrens Act') of 1868. The last named imposed a duty on landlords to keep houses in good repair. If they failed, the local authority had power to close the house or to carry out repairs at the owner's expense. The Torrens Act is the first of the innumerable housing laws passed by all parties during the last 100 years. It also established an entirely new concept, the right of the community to interfere with the sanctity of private property in the interest of public health.

These measures, especially the 1866 Sanitary Act, gave local authorities much greater power to abate nuisances and clean up the towns. But they still had no effective means of enforcement. After 1866 Simon became increasingly concerned with the inadequacy of public health supervision, both central and peripheral. Two central bodies controlled peripheral administration. The Poor Law Board, founded in 1847, was a Government Department. The Medical Department was directly responsible to the Privy Council, without ministerial representation in Parliament. This dichotomy resulted in a multiplicity of local authorities which seemed inevitably to increase with every new Act.

In 1868 Disraeli agreed to appoint a Commission of Enquiry. Disraeli fell from power but, in the following year, Gladstone appointed a Royal Commission to examine sanitary organization at central and peripheral levels. The main findings were accepted by government and opposition. The Commission instigated three important Acts. The Local Government Board Act, 1871, established a new government department, the Local Government Board, to which were transferred the powers and duties of the Poor Law Board and of the Medical Department of the Privy Council, thus ending the divided responsibility. The Public Health Act, 1872, virtually ended the old multi-parish system of local government by dividing the whole country, except London, into districts and placing each district under a single authority responsible for administering sanitary law. Every district was required to appoint a Medical Officer of Health and a Sanitary Inspector.

Thus in August 1871 John Simon ceased to be an official employed by the Privy Council and became Medical Officer of a new Government Department, the Local Government Board. During the next year he shared the work of drafting the last of the Commission's three Bills. Commonly called 'The Great Public Health Act' of 1875, this remarkable piece of legislation included in its scope almost all the recommendations made by Simon and his team. It covered sewerage, nuisances, offensive trades, adulterated and diseased foods, infectious disease, prevention of epidemics, foundation and inspection of infirmaries, cleaning and paving highways, housing, purchase of land for amenities, inspection of markets and slaughterhouses, imposition of sanitary regulations by local bye-law, among other matters. During the next sixty years, the 1875 Act permitted implementation of all the measures advocated by the sanitary reformers in the past forty years.

The Act was Simon's last major work. He lived to see Britain changed into a cleaner and more healthy land, its public health service the finest in the world, but he watched the advance from the touchline. The Local Government Board, which he had done so much to create, was a government department more concerned in its early years with Poor Law business than with public health. Simon the inspired leader became Simon the desk official. Laymen are always jealous of the specialist administrator. During the years 1871—6 the Medical Branch lost ground, becoming increasingly subservient to lay officials. In 1876 Simon found his power so eroded that his usefulness had almost gone. 'With extreme pain' he resigned after one final, fierce battle with the Treasury. He was followed in the post of Principal Medical Officer by three members of his old Privy Council team, E. C. Seaton 1876—9, George Buchanan 1879—92 and Richard Thorne Thorne 1892—9.

Governments and political parties have claimed credit for the magnificent public health system of modern Britain. Local authorities point to the salutary advances made under their beneficent rule. There are a host of men, doctors, lawyers, sanitary engineers and architects, who have helped to make a cleaner, healthier Britain. There have been enlightened governments and town councils—Liverpool is an example—and devoted medical officers, often working against intense local opposition. But in the history of public health there are two names which stand out above all others, two men who drove and persuaded government and local authority, medical profession and public alike to recognize the essential requirements of a city-dwelling populace.

Edwin Chadwick is not an attractive figure. An arrogant doctrinaire, his outlook was more that of a Nazi or a Fascist than a democratic Briton. His monument in the eyes of many social historians is the hated Union, the Poor Law Bastille. Yet the Union of the Guardians was not the Union envisaged by Chadwick and the workhouse has gone. Chadwick's eternal monument is the paved town, the clean street, the pure unfailing water supply and the drains which carry off our waste. John Simon is the antithesis of Edwin Chadwick. Chadwick loud-mouthed, bigoted, a dictator; Simon open-minded, a quiet scientist, diplomatic, a persuasive and inspiring leader. His memorial is the decent home, clean food, the prevention of industrial disease. Both were honoured with knighthoods, but the one was dismissed, the other forced to resign from high office. In remembering their names we should also spare a thought for Asiatic cholera, the fear of which shattered complacency and opened the public mind to the idea of sanitary reform.

Three major evils, alcohol, syphilis and tuberculosis, damaged the people of industrial Britain to an extent even greater than smallpox or cholera. Drinking to excess resulted in cruelty and neglect of children, a sordid home, unemployment, and too little money available for proper food. Untreated syphilis not only produced its dreadful terminal manifestations of tabes and general paralysis but infected the unborn child, giving rise to congenital blindness, deafness, idiocy and malformations. The 'ginnified urchin' of a Cruickshank or Hablot Browne illustration to a Dickens novel is a product of drink and syphilis as well as of poverty. Consumption, phthisis or pulmonary tuberculosis not only caused prolonged disabling illness but killed the wage-earner in his prime, leaving a widow and orphans to fend for themselves.

Alcoholism is a disease resulting from over-indulgence in an innocent escape upon which the subject becomes dependent. In this respect, alcohol resembles all other means of escape, whether smoking, fantasy-making or the taking of drugs. It is overindulgence in the escape, and not the means of escape itself, which is evil. This fact is not well understood today and was certainly not recognized a century ago. Social reformers warred against alcohol but failed to realize that dwellers in industrial towns turned to alcohol because they possessed no other means of escape from sordid conditions of life and work. This failure to provide any alternative to alcohol is the primary reason for heavy drinking in slum areas and industrial towns during the eighteenth and nineteenth centuries.

Alcohol cannot have been a major social problem in Britain until the seventeenth century. Beer was the staple drink of all classes. The first commercial brewery opened in 1492 but a far greater volume of liquor was produced in the home or the inn for many years to come. The brewer fined his beer with a bundle of twigs, removing as much as possible of the floating yeast, and preserved the 'bush' to provide a ferment for the next batch of wort. Except in wealthy houses, the resultant beer was drunk within a few days and direct from the vat, without intermediate barrelling. The thick muddy product always contained much free yeast and had a variable but generally low alcoholic content. It was food rather than drink and added some desirable vitamins to the diet of the predominantly meat eating baron as well as to that of the peasant who lived almost exclusively upon bread.

Chemists started to elaborate the method of fractional distillation early in the sixteenth century. The small quantities of spirit produced were medicines rather than substitutes for beer or wine. The names eau-de-vie and usquebaugh, both meaning water of life, remind us that brandy and whisky originated as cordials, preparations alleged to stimulate the heart's action. The Company of Distillers, which purveyed potable spirit, received its charter in 1638. The drinking of distilled spirit did not become popular in England until after the Battle of Ramillies in 1706. British troops developed a taste for Hollands, a Dutch spirit flavoured with juniper berries. Brandy and whisky could only be prepared from the distillate of fermented grape juice and grain or malt. Gin, a corruption of *genevre*, the French word for juniper, could be made from any spirit flavoured with juniper or turpentine. Distillers soon found that any fermentable material yielded a spirit which might be distributed to publicans who broke it with water and added flavouring. It was cheaper to ferment waste grain, vegetables of all kinds, rotten fruit and wood shavings, and to distil the spirit than to brew good ale. The distillate contained far more alcohol than wine or beer and, particularly when sawdust or woodshavings entered into the mixture, was more or less poisonous.

Over 5 million gallons of unbroken spirit, which had paid a duty of 2*d.* a gallon, were sold in England during 1735. No one can estimate the amount of illicit spirit produced. In 1736 the Government tried to check gin drinking by raising the tax, but the move produced rioting rather than decreased consumption. The problem had become so serious by 1751 that renewed action became essential. The Government again raised the tax and introduced laws forbidding retail sale by distillers and shopkeepers. A series of bad harvests in the years following 1780 did more to check spirit drinking than any legislation. Grain prices rose so high that distillation became unprofitable. The worst period had passed by 1790, but inordinately heavy drinking among all classes persisted until almost the end of the next century.

The non-conformist Churches, the Church of England Temperance Society, the Blue Ribbon Army, the Rechabites, Bands of Hope and the Salvation Army all fought against the scourge and demanded repressive legislation. Any legislation necessarily interfered with the liberty of the subject, a point made in a speech to the House of Lords in 1872 by Dr Magee, Bishop of Peterborough

> If I must take my choice whether England should be free or sober, I declare, strange as such a declaration may sound coming from one of my profession, that I should say it would be better that England should be free than that England should be compulsorily sober.

In view of opposition such as this, it is not surprising that the first Licensing Act did not enter the Statute Book until 1904. Amended by the Licensing Consolidation Act, 1910, legislation aimed at drastically reducing the number of public houses. Restricted opening hours were not introduced until the Defence of the Realm Act in 1915, which also forbade treating. By 1919 the tax on spirits had been increased to 36*s*. a gallon. These measures did much to decrease consumption, but force of public opinion played a greater part. Revulsion against drunkenness became apparent during the last two decades of the nineteenth century. Just as a fashion originating in the upper income group is gradually accepted by working-class homes, so overt intoxication became a social crime in all ranks of society. This had the curious and revealing consequence of weaning university undergraduates and gilded youth of the 1890s from overindulgence in alcohol to chain smoking of cigarettes and of ushering in the national Age of the Woodbine during the First World War.

We cannot assess the damage done by alcohol in the eighteenth and nineteenth centuries. Danger was greatly increased by prevalent malnutrition. The wealthy meat-eating class could drink far more with comparative safety than the poor who suffered from chronic protein deficiency. A low protein diet combined with alcoholic excess resulted in the more distressing manifestations, delirium tremens and cirrhosis of the liver. It is noticeable that the death rate for the whole of England actually outstripped the birth rate during the years 1722—38, although this was before gin drinking had reached its peak. In London, at the height of the gin era 1742—4, the number of burials doubled the number of baptisms. The appalling mortality of measles among young children during the mideighteenth century can be attributed indirectly to gin. Measles is not in itself a dangerous illness of childhood, always provided the patient is carefully nursed. Gin-sodden parents are unlikely to make good nurses. But there is little need to be specific. In general terms of preventible misery, poverty and degradation, alcohol has proved a dangerous friend to the working class.

Syphilis, the second great scourge of industrial Britain, has been exaggerated as to its incidence although not as to its evil effects. The Victorian aura of secrecy which shrouded prostitution and its accompanying infections tended to give the impression that venereal disease was rampant among the lower orders. There is no reason to suppose a lesser prevalence among the upper and middle classes. The Great Age of syphilis had passed before the rise of industrial towns. Introduced into Britain during the last decade of the fifteenth century, syphilis became one of the most common of all diseases during the sixteenth. But its reign as a virulent infection, transmitted by means other than coitus, was a short one. Henry VIII may have acquired his syphilis by means of a kiss (traditionally from Cardinal Wolsey) but the acute infection had settled to its present status as a chronic venereal disease before the reigns of Charles II, who probably suffered from it, and of James II who certainly did.* So

---

* The word 'certainly' must be modified by the phrase 'in the author's opinion'. No *certain* diagnosis can be made on second-hand evidence. Many historians, medical and lay, have challenged the view that syphilis

terrible may be the character changes produced in the terminal stage and so devastating the effects of these changes when the victim is in a position of power, that syphilis has undoubtedly altered the course of history from time to time. The connection between syphilis and its most dangerous manifestation, general paralysis of the insane, was not firmly established until 1913, although suspected for three-quarters of a century. Only of recent years have historians searched the records for earlier symptoms in a famous eccentric or notorious oppressor. Such researches tend to focus attention upon the mad cruelties which may follow infection of an individual. But these are rare incidents; the real tragedy of syphilis lies in the degeneration of whole families, whether they are highly placed or in humble circumstances.

Syphilis, like alcoholism, was primarily a disease of towns and the two are in some measure associated. Alcoholic loss of control favours promiscuity. The danger is particularly acute in garrison towns and naval stations where a number of healthy young men are herded together, the majority being unmarried. In the nineteenth century there were few outlets for energy and little opportunity for relaxation except the public house and the brothel. Brothels had no legal existence and were subject to no control. In France *'maisons de tolerance'* had been licensed since 1778 and registered prostitutes required to undergo fortnightly examination. Sweden and Denmark, the first countries to tackle venereal disease in a common-sense manner, instituted state-registered brothels in 1847 and 1874 respectively. No law existed in Britain until the Contagious Diseases Act of 1866. This applied only to garrison towns and naval stations. The Act required compulsory medical examination of prostitutes, who could be detained in a certified Lock hospital for three to six months if found to be suffering from venereal disease.

The Act is one of the more controversial in British legal history and aroused intense public opposition. A Royal Commission (1873) and a Select Committee of the House of Commons (1882) carefully examined its working and reported favourably. Such reports did not satisfy the public. In 1869 Mrs Josephine Butler, wife of the Principal of Liverpool College, founded the Ladies National Association for the Repeal of the Contagious Diseases Acts with the support of Florence Nightingale and Harriet Martineau among other highly-placed women. James Stansfield, President of the Poor Law Board, resigned his ministerial office in 1874 to help actively in the campaign. Working of the Act was suspended in 1883. Three years later Stansfield moved for repeal in the House of Commons and secured deletion of the Acts from the Statute Book in 1886.

---

was rife in the Tudor and Stuart families and have propounded alternative diagnoses. Such theories must command respect. The author maintains that the royal case-histories, personal, familial and obstetric, strongly indicate syphilis. The subject of Henry's ailments is discussed at some length in Cartwright and Biddiss, *Disease and History*, London, 1972.

At this distance of time it is a little difficult to understand the reasoning which lay behind such intense and sincere opposition. There can be no doubt that the campaigners believed it inhuman to enforce humiliating medical examination and confinement to hospital upon women. There is truth in the argument that legislation imputed 'sin' only to the female and not to the male. But we must question whether the underlying reason is not to be found in the strange Victorian attitude to sex. Every night hundreds of prostitutes solicited quite openly in respectable streets. Gentlemen of the very highest social rank maintained separate establishments for their mistresses while living blameless married lives and were not over secretive about it. Yet many parents of large families never saw each other naked and would have thought it shameful to do so. Many an Angelina embarked upon her wedding night with only the maternal advice 'You must do everything that dear Edwin tells you—remember, dearest child, *everything* that he tells you.' It was a queer mixture of intense sexual activity combined with the pretence that sexual action and appetite did not exist. By recognizing the existence of prostitution, the Acts offended Victorian morality. Since the Acts did little to check the spread of venereal disease, their repeal was not in itself a disaster. Far greater harm lay in the victory of secrecy. From 1886 until 1914 neither prostitution nor venereal disease officially existed in Britain and so no action could be taken.

Medical examinations during the South African War uncovered a deplorably low standard of physical fitness. Recruits, especially from industrial areas, were found to be undersized, of poor physique, and suffering from various preventible diseases and deformities. The revelation came as a jolting blow to the pride of a nation which believed itself divinely created to rule the earth. National arrogance refused to admit that a large proportion of the British population had been turned into chronic invalids by the very processes which made Britain the most wealthy and highly civilized nation in the world. Investigators tended to ignore the combination of evils which produced mass degeneration and tried to isolate a single cause. Syphilis was the obvious candidate. From 1903 onwards a number of medical and social workers conducted surveys, usually in a rather amateur fashion. They did good by bringing the problem into the open but there is no doubt that, since they were enthusiasts determined to find a single cause, they greatly exaggerated the incidence.

Two early twentieth-century discoveries profoundly affected the detection and treatment of syphilis. The complement fixation test, introduced by August von Wassermann in 1906, reveals the presence of infection even when the disease is quiescent, without apparent symptoms. Salvarsan, the famous '606' discovered by Paul Ehrlich and Sahachiro Hata in 1910, replaced the unpleasant and ineffectual treatment with mercury. These discoveries, coupled with some relaxation of the taboo surrounding discussion of venereal disease, induced the Local Government Board in 1913 to investigate the arrangements necessary for adequate large-scale treatment. A Royal Commission, set up on 1 November, was charged to explore the problem and recommend action, a special provision being that there should be no return to the type of legislation exemplified by the Contagious Diseases Acts.

The Scandinavian countries had actively and sensibly fought against venereal disease for over a century. As their legislation developed, four main requirements emerged. These are: notification of cases, compulsory treatment, strict anonymity, and the total banning of all quack remedies. The major difficulty is to combine notification with anonymity. The 1913 Royal Commission issued its report on 11 February 1916, at a time when venereal disease had enormously increased owing to the special conditions of warfare. The Commission recommended that local authorities be empowered to provide free diagnosis and treatment which should not be confined to residents of the area governed by the authority. This simple and sensible recommendation helped to preserve anonymity of the individual. The Commission could find no way of combining notification with strict anonymity and decided the latter to be essential. They advised entire prohibition of advertisements for remedies. The most important part of the report dealt with proper education in place of secrecy. The Commission advised recognition of a National Council for Combating Venereal Disease (later known as the British Social Hygiene Council) to be the authoritative body for spreading knowledge and giving advice. Special instruction should form an essential part of a medical student's course.

The Government accepted these proposals and found it possible to implement them under the 'great' Public Health Act, 1875. Clinics, usually attached to voluntary hospitals, came into operation in mid-1917. These formed the backbone of the service; in 1956, when the incidence of syphilis had greatly declined, there were still 229 clinics in England and Wales. Many local authorities posted the address of the nearest clinic in public urinals, a simple and common-sense method of advertisement. In 1922 the General Medical Council made regulations for teaching students. The most notable reform came in 1925 when local authorities were empowered to undertake a programme of education. Since education of this type can be achieved only by public discussion and overt acceptance that there is a matter to be discussed, the social taboo which overlaid the whole subject had at last been removed. Frank recognition of the public danger combined with anonymity of the individual removed a great deal both of fear and of stigma. This salutary change of approach did much to transform the patient, particularly when suffering the congenital type, from the sinner into the unfortunate.

Notification and compulsory treatment were widely advocated between the two World Wars, but general opinion regarded compulsion as an infringement of liberty and notification as a threat to anonymity. Persuasion was held preferable. Many VD clinics appointed social workers to investigate home problems. In 1925 a successful experiment in the port of Rotterdam suggested an extension of this work, first applied to Tyneside in Britain. Social workers not only ensured that sufferers were made aware of treatment facilities but also traced contacts and persuaded them to submit to Wassermann testing. This detection scheme was extended to the whole of Britain during the Second World War. At the same time the Government introduced notification and a certain measure of compulsion. Regulation 33B required any specialist in venereal disease to notify contacts to the Medical Officer of Health. The MOH had power to compel treatment if he received two or more notifications applying to any one person. In 1944, 8,339 contacts were notified, 3,696 of these traced, and 2,858 persuaded to undergo treatment, 827 being compelled after two or more notifications. Eighty-two were prosecuted for refusing treatment. The regulation ended in 1947, but the machinery for tracing contacts remained and social workers continued their invaluable task of investigation and persuasion. As in 1914—18, so in the Second World War the incidence of venereal disease greatly increased. The measures taken, combined with a much more effective means of treatment in the antibiotic penicillin, produced a very rapid fall during the post-war years until syphilis had been apparently defeated in 1956 and clinics were rapidly closing for lack of patients. It is a terrible reflection upon modern society that the magnificent work done between 1917 and 1956 has failed to stamp out this totally unnecessary disease. Partly by the emergence of a penicillin resistant organism, partly by introduction of a more virulent strain through immigration, but mainly because of a laxer moral code and sheer carelessness among young people, syphilis is again one of our social problems.

From the tragic theme of syphilis we pass to the third of our scourges, tuberculosis, and here the story has a happier ending. Tuberculosis is a disease more ancient than man, caused by an organism which is perhaps the oldest living creature on earth. Certain primitive cold-blooded animals are infected with saprophytic organisms, normally living on dead tissue. These somewhat resemble the bacillus of tuberculosis and produce 'tuberculoid' changes in cold-blooded animals. They also produce changes rather similar to tuberculosis when injected into warm-blooded animals. The inference is that there has been a gradual adaptation of a saprophytic organism from dead tissue to living, from cold-blooded to warm-blooded animals, and so to the human.

Part of this theory is borne out by the great prevalence of tuberculosis among animals. Five types of bacillus are recognized but we are concerned only with the bovine and human types. Man can be infected by both. The bovine type, usually acquired by drinking milk from tuberculous cows, tends to be a disease of childhood. The human type, usually acquired by direct spread from one person to another, tended until quite recently to be a disease of the young adult. Tuberculosis can affect every bodily structure. The bovine type more commonly affected glands, joints or bones, and was known as scrofula or the King's Evil; the human type more often attacked the lungs and was known as phthisis or consumption. An attack of the bovine type protects the patient against infection by the human type. Being almost confined to children, the bovine infection could be an actual safeguard against more serious illness in later life. Although a number of children developed an illness resulting in death or crippling deformity, many showed nothing more than an enlarged gland or a slight temperature. They had been infected by the bovine bacillus but their natural resistance had been sufficient to overcome the very small invasion. This 'attack' was sufficient to protect against further infection by the bovine type *and also against the human type*. The importance of this fact must be emphasized. In closely packed communities, human invasion was likely to be far more massive and far more difficult to resist; the immunity conferred by the bovine type was therefore advantageous. In the years of high incidence of tuberculosis many doctors, especially in Britain, believed that treatment of milk to render it free of tubercle bacilli carried a danger because, although such treatment might save the lives of some children, it would place many more at risk through later and almost inevitable contact with a human source.

Evidence of tuberculous infection is to be found from the earliest times, in the tombs of Egypt and in American skeletons dating from the pre-Columban era. One of the most interesting of medical discoveries is the body of a 21st dynasty Ammonite priest named Nesperehan who died about 1000 BC. He not only shows the typical hunch-back appearance (kyphosis) of advanced spinal tuberculosis but also the cavity formed in the lower part of the abdomen above the hip-joint which would now be known as a psoas abscess. The Hippocratic texts record recognizable symptoms and appearances. Aretaeus of Alexandria, writing in the second century AD, described the classical *habitas phthisica* 'the slender, with prominent throats, whose shoulder blades protrude like wings, who are pale and have narrow chests'. All civilizations, all countries, have been ravaged by tuberculosis. Physicians have attempted cures in all ages. The Hindus advised out-door living, exercise, and sleeping in goat stables. Galen taught that the disease is contagious and warned against contact with infected persons. He sent his patients to Stabia, a resort on the coast of Italy opposite the Isle of Capri. Rhazes and Avicenna of the mediaeval Arabian school recommended draughts of asses' milk and powdered crab shells. The latter provided additional calcium, a treatment revived in the late nineteenth century.

Magic or miraculous cure played its part and took a strange form. The King's Evil or scrofula, commonly affecting the glands of the neck, was supposed to respond to the Royal Touch. Touching is a very ancient custom, dating back at least to Clovis the Frank in AD 496. French kings regularly touched until 1775 and the custom was resurrected by Charles X, an ardent believer in the Divine Right, when he ascended the throne of France in 1824. Edward the Confessor seems to have been responsible for introducing touching to England, and the practice was followed by all his successors until 1714. Charles II touched in exile and dealt with 6,275 sufferers in the year of his restoration. By the time of his death in 1683 he had touched no less than 92,107 people. History does not relate how many he cured, but the figure suggests a high incidence of glandular tuberculosis in the seventeenth century. William III continued the ceremony, but had little faith in it for he accompanied each touching with the words 'God grant you better health and more sense'. Queen Anne touched no less a person than the two-year-old Samuel Johnson in 1711–12. Johnson must have been one of the last subjects of this curious tradition, for George I abolished the rite when he came to the throne in 1714 and it was never revived.

The early history of the pulmonary form in Britain is not clear. Some historians hold that consumption was a disease of the well-nourished upper class rather than of the under-privileged until the eighteenth century. They point to the interesting medical history of the Tudor dynasty as an example. Edward VI died of tuberculosis and hereditary syphilis, a combination not uncommon among nineteenth century slum children. Edward's illegitimate half-brother, the Duke of Richmond, died of a long-standing lung complaint at seventeen. Their grandfather, Henry VII, died of 'tissic', usually considered an old term for consumption, in 1509, while his son Arthur, brother of Henry VIII, died of the same complaint in 1502. But deaths of notabilities attracted attention, whereas deaths of lesser persons did not. It is equally logical to infer from 'the royal case-history' that pulmonary tuberculosis was widespread, attacking all classes including the most highly privileged. This must have been true of late seventeenth-century towns, for John Locke wrote in 1685 that one-fifth of all deaths in London were caused by consumption.

Nor is it safe to argue that an open-air life with ample supplies of wholesome food protected our forebears of the Agricultural Age. The rosy countryman in his flower-decked cottage is a myth. The truth is a squalid village inhabited by half-starved, crowded families. Such conditions provided an excellent medium for the tubercle bacillus. But, although whole families might be infected, the considerable distances between villages tended to isolate foci of disease. Such is not true of the town, where close-packed dwellings permitted easy spread from one family to another. The bovine type must have been more common in rural areas and, although the cause of crippling disease and death, also offered some protection. Again, the agricultural labourer at least worked in clean air and in comparative segregation. Not so the factory operative, often just as badly fed and housed as the countryman, but working in crowded conditions and an enclosed, contaminated atmosphere. It is the rise of the town and the Industrial Revolution which gave tuberculosis mastery over Western Europe and North America.

The virtually unchallenged reign of tuberculosis lasted from the third quarter of the eighteenth century until the Second World War. During this period of 150 years it became far more common among the under-privileged than among the privileged, although the latter suffered severely by modern standards. Tuberculosis was regarded as synonymous with poverty. Although true, this is not the whole truth. The present view is that poor living and working conditions, combined with inadequate diet, do not wholly account for the high incidence. The rise in mortality from tuberculosis during all major wars may be partly due to these causes but suggests that physical and psychological strain also play a part. This concept of 'strain' is supported by an increased prevalence of tuberculosis among pregnant women employed in industry. Nineteenth century industrial towns lacked those amenities supposed to lessen risk of infection: fresh air, sunlight, adequate leisure, proper facilities for personal hygiene. The sum of these inadequacies cannot entirely account for the high incidence during the nineteenth century, because all had existed in earlier towns. The new factors were exacerbation of previous evils, gross overcrowding in home and factory, and acute strain consequent on overwork and the nagging fear of losing the means of livelihood.

We cannot attempt to estimate the number of people affected by tuberculosis of one form or another. We have already inferred that the disease was widespread at the end of the seventeenth century. John Brownlee, investigating the relative incidence of infections, believed that the highest death rate in London occurred about 1800 and that provincial industrial towns reached their zenith a few years later. If this be so, mortality at the beginning of the nineteenth century must have been very high. Accurate figures are available from the introduction of death registration in 1838. During the first five years, 1838—43, the pulmonary form, consumption, caused an annual average of 60,000 deaths. The number then fell slowly. In 1851—5, pulmonary tuberculosis caused 51,000 deaths annually and the slow fall continued until the First World War. Stated in terms of deaths per thousand of the population, the figures are 3.6 in 1851, 1.9 in 1900, 1.4 in 1916. Consumption every year killed more people in nineteenth-century Britain than smallpox, scarlet fever, measles, whooping cough and typhus fever put together. Pulmonary tuberculosis was by far the greater killer; other forms added less than 10,000 deaths a year. But in the latter part of the nineteenth century a very high proportion of surgical operations were performed on account of tuberculosis of glands, bones and joints. In 1889—90 surgery of tuberculosis accounted for 26 per cent of operations and the proportion still stood at 20.5 per cent in 1901.

A killer such as this challenged doctors to find an efficient means of treatment but, as in the case of all disease, little progress could be made until the cause had been found. The idea that consumption is contagious dates from very early times; not until 1865 did Jean Antoine Villemin, a young French army surgeon, actually prove that it could be transmitted to animals by inoculation. In the preceding year Louis Pasteur propounded the Germ Theory. In 1882 Robert Koch, a general practitioner of Wollstein in Germany, isolated the tubercle bacillus. Over eighty more years passed before an efficient means of attacking the bacillus could be found. Attempts to use ordinary antiseptics failed because the organisms lay deep in the lungs and could not be reached without damaging the tissues. Treatment by vaccines prepared from tubercle bacilli also failed. Tuberculin or 'Koch's fluid', first prepared by E. L. Trudeau in 1890 and a little later by Koch, proved not only useless but actively dangerous. But tuberculin is an important step forward, because it provided a simple means of skin testing. The test demonstrates whether or not a person has already suffered a minor tuberculous infection and so whether he is still susceptible.

Until the Second World War, treatment of tuberculosis depended upon good food, sunlight, fresh air and rest. In 1796 John Coakley Lettsom, a Quaker physician, founded an institution at Margate, Kent, for thirty-six children suffering from scrofula; this became known as the Royal Sea Bathing Hospital. George Boddington, a Birmingham doctor, opened a small hospital for consumptives at Sutton Coldfield in 1843, but his fresh-air treatment encountered so much opposition that he was forced to abandon the project. Hermann Brehmer, a physician, started a sanatorium at Göbersdorf, Silesia, in 1859; Peter Dettweiller, who had been one of Brehmer's patients, built a similar institution at Falkenstein in 1876. The most famous and influential of these early sanatoria is that founded by Edward Livingstone Trudeau in 1884. Trudeau himself suffered from consumption. He planned a number of small separate cottages surrounding a central laboratory where he conducted his investigations. His sanatorium, situated at Saranac Lake in the healthy Adirondack Mountains of USA, formed the prototype of many others.

By 1911 eighty-four sanatoria of this type provided 8,000 beds in Britain. They had been established and were largely maintained by voluntary effort; local authorities provided or paid for only one-fifth of the beds. Lloyd George's Insurance Act of 1911 is commonly regarded as the first attempt by the State to interfere in the treatment of disease. The Act provided £1.5 million for the erection of sanatoria. The Local Government Board encouraged county councils to apply for capital grants from the fund, and a number of new institutions were opened. The incidence of tuberculosis was already falling quite rapidly in 1911 but the First World War checked the fall because overwork and a lowered standard of nutrition combined with strain to increase both incidence and mortality. The fall resumed after the war, but did not keep pace with the number of sanatoria available. In 1930 500 institutions provided 25,000 beds but many patients suffering from active pulmonary tuberculosis still had to be nursed in their own homes.

Attempts to prevent tuberculosis helped to reduce mortality in the nineteenth century. As early as 1567 Paracelsus drew attention to the relation between pulmonary disease and mining. In 1799 Thomas Beddoes of Bristol noted that brassworkers and stonecutters were unusually prone to consumption. Gradually it became recognized that dusty trades, particularly when the dust is from silica, placed workers at special risk. From 1870 onwards Britain introduced a number of regulations and parliamentary Acts designed to protect workers in dusty employments. Compulsory wearing of masks, wetting of material, ventilation of factories, and the substitution of limestone for silicaceous abrasives were some of the measures. A most beneficial advance accidentally occurred during an attempt to produce synthetic diamonds when Edward G. Acheson of

Pennsylvania prepared the harmless and efficient abrasive carborundum. About 1870 A. C. Gerlach proved that tuberculosis can be carried by milk. In 1873 Edward Klebs showed that such milk is produced from cows which are themselves infected. Theobald Smith of Harvard University isolated the responsible bacillus, the bovine type, in 1898. Smith showed that the bovine bacillus, although differing from the human, will cause tuberculosis in man. In 1901 Robert Koch muddled the issue by stating that the human bacillus cannot produce tuberculosis in cattle. His finding partly stimulated formation of a Royal Commission on Tuberculosis, largely composed of well-known scientists. The Commission carried out experiments from 1901 until 1914 on a farm at Stansted loaned by Sir James Blyth. By 1904 they had proved that the human type produced in cattle a disease identical with that caused by the bovine type. In 1907 the Commission reported that cow's milk infected with bovine tubercle bacilli is a cause of tuberculosis in man and that a very large proportion of tuberculosis contracted by ingestion resulted from a bovine source. They stressed the urgent need to prevent sale of infected milk.

Louis Pasteur had shown that souring of milk is due to a micro-organism. He proved that heated milk will not sour if sealed from the air. In 1880 the German firm of Ashborn manufactured the first commercial apparatus for the 'pasteurization' of milk. The purpose was simply to delay souring. At the end of the nineteenth century scientists became interested in pasteurization as a means of destroying harmful micro-organisms. Dr Charles E. North of New York introduced a low tempera-ture pasteurizing plant in 1907 which rapidly came into general use throughout the United States. North submitted milk to a temperature of $140°-150°F$ for at least thirty minutes and immediately cooled it to $55°F$. Not only did the process kill disease-producing microorganisms, including the tubercle bacillus, but it delayed souring and was therefore commercially desirable.

Meanwhile, Theobald Smith's work suggested an attempt to eliminate tuberculosis from dairy herds. This is comparatively simple, for cattle can be submitted to the tuberculin test and any infected animals slaughtered. But it is also very expensive. In 1917 about 16 per cent of dairy cattle in USA and 25 per cent in Britain were estimated to be tuberculous. That year the United States Bureau of Animal Husbandry started a programme of eradication, supported by government funds for compensation. A combination of pasteurization and Tuberculin Tested herds reduced the incidence of tuberculosis among American children to about half that obtaining in Britain at the equivalent date. Britain did not take strenuous action until 1922, when the Peoples' League of Health reported that no less than 40 per cent of dairy cows suffered from tuberculosis. Infected milk was actively secreted by 0.2 per cent of these. Examination of raw milk from various districts revealed tubercle bacilli in from 2—13 per cent of samples. The danger was much greater than these figures suggest, because one actively tuberculous cow will infect the milk collected in bulk from a number of farms. The Ministry of Health therefore issued the first Milk (Special Designation) Order which required all milk to be described as *Pasteurized* or *Tuberculin Tested and Pasteurized*. The latter might contain milk obtained only from tuberculosis-free herds.

Pasteurization and tuberculin testing, particularly the latter, greatly reduced the incidence of the form affecting glands, bones and joints. The incidence of phthisis or consumption remained high. Since spread is by droplet infection, one infected person can transmit tuberculosis to all the members of a household, just as a common cold will generally infect the whole family. This raises a grave social problem, for the wage-earning head of the household is endangered. Consumption is rarely a swiftly killing disease, more usually causing a prolonged illness whether the outcome is death or recovery. Thus the wage earner, particularly if in heavy work, will be unable to support himself or his family for months or even years. Purely from the economic viewpoint, a working class family is better off if the wage earner is dead than if he is a chronic invalid, unable to work and requiring support. It follows that a single case of consumption may result in disaster. There is urgent need to isolate the first case, to examine the rest of the family at frequent intervals, and to provide a job within the capacity of the sick wage earner, or else to support him and his dependants.

The concept of pulmonary tuberculosis as a familial catastrophe was first understood by Thomas Beddoes who founded his Preventive Medical Institution at Little Tower Court, a Bristol slum area, in 1803. His *Rules* make clear that he purposed to examine not only the sick patient but the seemingly healthy members of the family. He hoped to detect infection at the earliest possible moment 'to check the canker of disease as soon as it fastens on the frame and by degrees to root it out'. This brilliant eccentric was far ahead of his time. Both his patients and the medical profession suspected his motives and his Institution failed, although it survived for ten years after Beddoes' death in 1808. A more successful pioneer of the 'social approach' is Robert Philip, an Edinburgh physician, who founded the Victoria Dispensary for Consumption in 1887. Philip's principle is similar to that of Beddoes. He taught the need to consider the whole family as the unit of investigation, his object being to determine the presence of infection not only in the obviously consumptive patient but in apparently unaffected members of the household. Thus he started the tracing of tuberculous contacts. Philip also campaigned for notification, isolation, sanatorium care of the sick, and provision of colonies to provide light work. He envisaged his dispensary as a central agency from which all these functions could be organized.

The first English dispensary started work on Philip's lines at Paddington in 1909. Oxfordshire and Sheffield followed in 1910 and 1911. The number rose to sixty-four shortly after the Lloyd George Act, but only fourteen were provided by local authorities. The remaining fifty owed their foundation and maintenance to voluntary effort, stimulated by the National Association for the Prevention of Tuberculosis formed in

1898. The Education Act, 1907, provided for medical examination of school children at regular intervals and thus helped in the early recognition of disease. Notification was at first voluntary and local, the earliest town to require notification being Oldham, Lancs, in 1897, but became compulsory in 1911. This greatly assisted Medical Officers of Health in their search for contacts. The Public Health Act, 1913, was particularly aimed at tuberculosis. It required county councils to prepare schemes for prevention and treatment. A scheme implied appointment of a Tuberculosis Officer, nurses for home visiting, a voluntary after-care committee, and the provision of dispensaries and sanatoria.

The First World War interrupted this steady advance but saw the institution of a quite new form of endeavour. The problem of 'light open-air work' and of rehabilitation had never been tackled. In 1914 Pendrill Charles Varrier-Jones sought the advice of Sir Clifford Allbutt, a leading physician, on the subject and in 1916 opened a small village settlement which later moved to Papworth in Cambridgeshire. The settlement consisted of a number of residential cottages, a sanatorium and hospital, and workshops. Selected tuberculous patients were admitted with their families to live in the cottages for an indefinite period and to work in the shops under strict medical supervision. Similar institutions opened at Barrowmoor, Wrenbury Hall and Preston Hall. These village settlements enabled a stabilized tuberculous patient to live with his family and undertake work within his capacity, thus averting the tragedy of the patient, seemingly cured and in good health, returning to an unsuitable job and suffering a relapse. Varrier-Jones hoped the settlements would be self-supporting but all required financial help. Although the scheme failed in this respect and so never became widespread, the underlying idea gave rise to the modern rehabilitation centre. In 1943 the Government established special factories to provide light work (Remploy) and in 1944 employers of more than twenty workers were required to take a quota of 3 per cent of disabled persons. The quota included people suffering from arrested or quiescent tuberculosis.

The terms 'quiescent' and 'arrested' suggest advances in treatment of the disease. Attempts to cure tuberculosis have been made for many years. The most hopeful seemed to be rest and this was applied to the affected lung by surgical means. In 1821 James Carson, an English physician, advocated filling the afflicted side of the thorax with air, thus collapsing the lung and permitting it to rest, but his idea was not put into practice until the 1880s. 'Artificial pneumothorax' had been induced in about 400 cases before 1910. The procedure became far more popular after the First World War when experience with battle casualties showed that useful existence is possible with only one lung. Another method, section or crushing of the phrenic nerve supplying the diaphragm, was suggested by Ferdinand Sauerbruch of Griefswald, Germany, in 1913 but again did not come into common use until after 1918. Between the wars attempts were sometimes made to remove infected lobes of the lung or even the whole lung, but such procedures were both difficult and dangerous until controlled respiration, introduced into anaesthesia during the Second World War, permitted the surgeon to operate on a more or less immobile chest.

Many workers tried to produce a safe and efficient vaccine. We have already noted that Koch's tuberculin proved too dangerous for use in prevention or cure. In 1902 Emil Adolf von Behring of Marburg prepared 'bovovaccine', an attenuated strain of human bacilli with which he hoped to stamp out tuberculosis in cattle. This also proved to be dangerous, but is probably the starting point of the famous or notorious 'Spahlinger treatment' which had a great vogue and caused an equally great controversy in the years 1921–35. Henri Spahlinger described his preparation as anti-tuberculous serum, but a good deal of mystery surrounds both the serum and its inventor. In 1906 Leon Charles Albert Calmette and his colleague at the Pasteur Institute in Paris, Camille Guerin, started work on von Behring's idea of using an alien tubercle bacillus. Unlike von Behring, they sought a cure for human tuberculosis by use of a bovine strain. They cultured and subcultured a selected strain on a medium containing glycerin and ox bile. The patience of the true research worker is well demonstrated by the fact that Calmette made 231 subcultures, each at an interval of three weeks, over a period of thirteen years before satisfying himself that he possessed an attenuated and permanently stabilized strain. Calmette, now working in Lille, continued his experiments during the 1914–18 war. Lille had been occupied by the Germans, who requisitioned all cattle. Calmette experimented with pigeons. His possession of numerous pigeons aroused suspicion and he narrowly escaped being shot as a spy.

Bacille-Calmette-Guerin or BCG, when injected into calves, caused a slight fever which cleared spontaneously without signs of tuberculosis. Used experimentally in 1921–4 it proved effective as a preventive vaccine in both cattle and infants. Calmette distributed a free supply to doctors and midwives in 1924, wisely cautioning that his preparation was only suitable for very young children. By the end of 1925 1,317 infants had been treated. Of these 586 had been in contact with tuberculosis. Six children died of the disease within six months of injection. These fatalities caused mistrust but vaccination with BCG continued to be used in France and gradually spread to other countries. In 1930 there occurred the frightful Lübeck disaster in Germany. Two hundred and thirty infants were inoculated from a single batch of BCG vaccine; of these, 173 developed tuberculosis and 68 died within a very short time. A court of enquiry decided that the culture of BCG received from the Pasteur Institute had either been contaminated or replaced by a lethal human strain. The chief physician to the general hospital and the head of Lübeck health department were found guilty of negligence and sentenced to terms of imprisonment. Despite this verdict, the reason for the tragedy has never been satisfactorily explained.

BCG did not again come into wide use until after the Second World War, when better laboratory control and standardization had virtually made such accidents impossible. World literature shows that by 1963 over

150 million BCG vaccinations were performed with only four deaths resulting. Britain, one of the last countries to adopt the method, estimated that between 1956 and 1963 tuberculosis developed at the rate of 1.9 per 1,000 untreated infants and at 0.40 per 1,000 when treated with BCG. Vaccination reduced incidence by 79 per cent. Protection lasted from seven to ten years and it was therefore important to revaccinate.

Direct attack upon tubercle bacilli became possible in 1948. Penicillin, the first antibiotic drug, proved ineffective against the organism but stimulated research for a similar weapon. In 1944 Salman Waksman of New Jersey, USA, isolated the antibiotic Streptomycin from the mould *Streptomyces griseus*, found growing in the throats of chickens in a heavily manured field. Streptomycin, lethal to the tubercle bacillus, was introduced into medicine in 1948. Unfortunately streptomycin-resistant strains emerged. Professor William Hugh Feldman worked on the problem in the University of Minnesota and found that a course of streptomycin can be combined with two drugs, para-aminosalicylic acid (PAS) and isonicotinic acid hydrazide (isoniazid) with excellent effect and, apparently, without danger of producing resistant strains.

The period of the Second World War saw another great advance. From 1939 to 1942 there was a shortlived rise in the incidence and mortality of tuberculosis. The rise was checked largely because the Government recognized the urgent need to maintain the tuberculosis service despite the heavy demand of warfare upon manpower. Wilhelm Conrad Röntgen of Würzburg in Germany discovered X-rays in 1895. Radiography proved of great value in detecting tuberculous lesions of the lung. As methods improved and as experience grew, lesions could be observed at an earlier stage and, finally, before any symptoms or clinical signs of disease appeared. Simplification of apparatus made possible the use of mobile units for mass radiography. The first of these operated in Lancashire in October 1943; fifteen units were at work by March 1945. Mass radiography revealed an unsuspected incidence of tuberculosis in the civilian population. If we take 250,000 as the number of known cases, then another 150,000 were added by mass radiography. The obvious difficulty is to persuade a wage-earner who suffers from no symptoms to give up his job and undergo treatment. The Government therefore provided a sum of up to £1 million for compensation in addition to ordinary sickness benefit. This measure, together with Remploy factories and the disabled persons scheme, helped to solve the problem.

Detection of susceptible persons by means of a modernized tuberculin test, BCG vaccine prepared under strict control, radiological examination, and the use of drugs are the weapons with which tuberculosis is fought. World Health Organization launched an immense campaign after the Second World War. Some idea of the magnitude of the effort to stamp out tuberculosis on a global scale can be gained from the fact that nearly 400 million people were tuberculin tested and 180 million vaccinated between 1948 and 1966. The effect upon the mortality in Britain can be seen from the following figures. In 1937, 27,754 people died and in 1949 the number for the first time fell below 20,000. Thereafter the rate of fall became increasingly steep, through 10,585 in 1952 and 8,902 in 1953 to 2,282 in 1965 and 2,354 in 1966.

No single medical advance has caused this dramatic decline, nor has the defeat of tuberculosis been due to medicine alone. The victory has been won by a combination of medical and scientific discoveries, social legislation, and improved amenities. Better housing, adequate nutrition, opportunity for relaxation, and good working conditions have all played a part. But we ought not to be complacent for there may be another and more decisive factor. The incidence and mortality of tuberculosis were already falling before improvement in living conditions or scientific discoveries could exert any effect. High family morbidity suggested a hereditary disposition, which the nineteenth century doctor called the 'tuberculous diathesis', a familial lack of resistance. Modern epidemiologists believe that familial *resistance* was more valid than familial *lack*. The resistance was hereditary, a gene handed down from parent to offspring. Since pulmonary tuberculosis is spread by droplet infection through coughing, speaking, or sneezing, a non-resistant family must easily acquire the disease from one casually infected member, but this would not be the case in a resistant family. Since mortality from consumption was high, a non-resistant family rapidly decreased in number, while the resistant family increased in the ordinary manner. If we accept the general opinion that incidence and mortality were at their peak shortly after 1800, then the fall during the first half of the nineteenth century can have been due only to the increasing emergence of genetic resistance. Natural phasing-out of non-resistant families continued until the Second World War, with social and medical interference gradually playing a larger part.

After the Second World War much improved methods of diagnosis, prevention by BCG vaccination, and direct treatment by surgery or drugs produced a very steep decline until the terrible scourge of tuberculosis was transformed into a disease less lethal and less prevalent than the 'trivial' illness of influenza. Of the three major evils which afflicted the industrial town, tuberculosis is today the one most certainly under control.

8 The birth of scientific medicine

Bubonic plague disappeared from Europe rather mysteriously and certainly not as the result of any medical advance. Smallpox began to decline before the introduction of preventive vaccination. Tuberculosis had already become a much less common disease before the discovery of an efficient treatment. Cholera and typhoid fever were beaten by sanitation and clean water supply rather than by drugs. These indisputable facts have suggested that medicine has played little part in the production of a comparatively healthy community. This thesis can, to a certain extent, be supported by population figures. In Chapter 6 we mentioned a swiftly rising population as one cause of the evils which marked the early years of the Industrial Age. A rather more detailed consideration of the subject may help us to decide whether the major medical and scientific advances of the nineteenth century did or did not benefit the general health of the nation.

The population of England and Wales has been estimated at about 4 million in 1300, at 2.1 million in 1377, and at just over 5 million in 1700. It probably took some 200 years for the population to recover from the Black Death, that is the 1300 figure of 4 million was not reached until the middle of the sixteenth century. Population continued to increase over the next 150 years, adding rather more than 1 million inhabitants to England and Wales, until in 1700 the low figure of 1377 had been more than doubled. We may therefore say that population doubled in a little more than three centuries. In 1851 the population of England and Wales was 18 million. In the decade 1725—35 the death rate actually outstripped the birth rate, and there must have been a fall in population at this time. It is therefore a safe assumption that the population of England and Wales quadrupled, or almost quadrupled, between 1735 and 1850, a period of 115 years or less than half the time between the Black Death and 1700. This large increase occurred despite the fact that towns were growing during the whole period 1735—1850 and the town lived upon the countryman. For the death rate in towns was in general greater than the live birth rate. The town population could only grow by fresh imports from the country.

No accurate information is available until the first census of 1801, but there is little doubt that the rising population was caused by a falling death rate. The number of live births must have slightly exceeded the number of deaths until 1725 in order to produce the increase. From 1725 until 1735 deaths exceeded the number of births. It has been estimated that the gap between the two figures then swiftly widened, from a birth rate of 33.3 per 1,000 and a death rate of 31.7 per 1,000 in 1740, through 33.3 per 1,000 and 26.7 per 1,000 in 1760, to 33.84 per 1,000 births and 19.98 per 1,000 deaths in 1820. From 1740 until 1760 very few, if any, more babies were being born but considerably fewer people were dying. After 1760 there is a slight increase in the birth rate and a very marked fall in the death rate. In fact, the maximum decennial increase, accurately revealed by the census returns, probably occurred in the decade 1811–21. The increase in these years was 18.06 per cent; thereafter the decennial increase slowly fell although total population continued to rise.

How are these figures to be interpreted? The phenomenon was not confined to Britain, but was general throughout Europe. In the opinion of G. M. Trevelyan (*English Social History*)

> The advance in population represented a rather larger birth rate and a very much reduced death rate. The survival of many more infants and the prolongation of the average life of adults mark off modern times from the past, and this great change began in the Eighteenth Century. It was due mainly to improved medical service.

But, one is entitled to ask, what improved medical service was this great change due to? We can discover no medical advance made in the eighteenth century, or any more efficacious treatment of disease, or any better care of the sick, that can possibly have resulted in a large-scale improvement of national health. Provision of hospitals touched very few people, and it is doubtful if hospital care prolonged life. Vaccination lay in the future and no disease had been conquered. Only plague had disappeared—seventy years before population started on its spectacular rise—and variolation may have done something to reduce mortality from smallpox during the latter half of the eighteenth century. But smallpox still caused many deaths and it seems that mortality from tuberculosis was on the increase.

'The survival of many more infants' is hypothetical. Registration of births did not start until 1837 and was not compulsory until 1874. Infant mortality, the number of children dying within a year of birth, is supposed to have stood at 250 per 1,000 in the mid-eighteenth century and to have fallen to 150 per 1,000 by 1850. But this is only supposition. In the four-year period 1876–80, infant mortality was 145 per 1,000, but it actually rose to an annual average of 153 per 1,000 during the decade of the 1890s. The steep fall did not begin until after 1905. Disregarding any medical advances, we know that there was considerable improvement in social hygiene during the last quarter of the nineteenth century. It is very difficult to accept the great fall of 100 per 1,000 during the century 1750–1850 if the real improvements of the late nineteenth century effected no further decrease.

We therefore cannot accept Professor Trevelyan's opinion that population growth 'was due mainly to improved medical service' and must look for some other explanation. Possibly this may be found in the great agricultural progress which became evident in the eighteenth century. The most momentous discovery, and that which radically changed the national diet, is the growing of crops for winter feed. Until the introduction of plentiful fodder, only breeding cattle could be kept through the winter months. The remainder were slaughtered in autumn and the meat salted. Some fresh meat, a larger supply of vegetables, and more milk in winter may have reduced the *childhood* rather than the *infant* mortality. Perhaps Lord Townshend's turnips should be accorded the major credit.

But there may be another explanation. Increase may have been due to removal of a population check which began to operate in the early sixteenth century and started to lessen its effect at the beginning of the eighteenth. There is some evidence that this may have occurred. If we take the baptized children of English monarchs, we find:

(a) From William the Conqueror until Henry VII (1066—1509) there were baptized sixty-nine infants of whom sixty survived into adult life and nine died before puberty.

(b) From Henry VIII until George I (1509—1727) there were baptized forty-six infants of whom twenty-one survived into adult life and twenty-five died before puberty.

(c) From George II until Victoria (1727—1901) there were baptized thirty-seven infants of whom thirty-four survived into adult life and three died before puberty.

T. H. Hollingsworth, in *A Demographic Study of the British Ducal Families*, investigated the percentage of male offspring who survived the first twenty years of life, and the percentage of female offspring who survived the first fifteen. His results may be tabulated:

Period	Males (%)	Females (%)
1330—1479	67	88
1480—1729	58	67
1730—1879	76	86

Hollingsworth is careful to point out that the period 1330—1479 may be affected by incomplete records, but his figures for ducal families tend to support those of the monarchy. Taken together, the two pieces of evidence suggest a higher mortality of young people in the period 1500—1730 than in either the preceding or succeeding years. In other words, some check upon ability to reach adult life operated during the sixteenth and seventeenth centuries.

We can postulate the nature of this check. Syphilis entered Europe at the end of the fifteenth century as a disease far more infectious than today. Smallpox seems to have been of a mild type until the sixteenth century. That mysterious illness known as the English Sweat, possibly a type of influenza, appeared in 1485, caused recurrent and lethal epidemics, and seems to have died out about 100 years later. Thus the sixteenth century was an age of new infections and the most telling of these may have been syphilis in its congenital form, since this causes not only miscarriages and stillbirths but also a large destruction of young people. The English Sweat either disappeared for no known reason or receded into an illness indistinguishable from 'ordinary influenza', and the latter is the more likely conjecture. The same probably happened in the case of smallpox, although here variolation may have helped. A similar argument can be applied to syphilis, for there is evidence that it was not so prevalent in the seventeenth century as in the sixteenth. Lessened virulence of three killing diseases such as are these, either through attenuation of the causative organism or by gradual development of mass resistance, must have permitted many more people to survive into adult life. Here, then is a possible explanation, or partial explanation, of the population increase which began in the eighteenth century.

Population continued to rise during the latter part of the nineteenth century. But this increase now becomes very remarkable. During the whole period 1740–1850, the birth rate showed a tendency to rise, reaching a peak of 35.44 per 1,000 in 1800. After 1876 the number of births started to fall rather steeply and stood at only 28.2 per 1,000 in 1900, a lower figure than in 1730 when deaths exceeded births. The population of England and Wales was 23 million in 1876 and 32 million in 1900. Thus many more people must have been surviving for much longer. Deaths fell particularly steeply in the towns; after 1870 average expectation of life was rather longer in industrial cities than in agricultural districts.

We certainly cannot claim that this improvement in health, particularly in the health of towns, resulted from medical discoveries alone. Progress had been made in a number of fields. Rapid communications rendered travel cheaper and gave opportunity for relaxation. Municipal authorities provided open spaces and means of leisure in museums and art galleries. Plentiful imports of cheap food ensured adequate nutrition. Hours of work were reduced and factory conditions bettered. Sanitation and water supply had been greatly improved. All these helped to build a healthier and therefore a longer lived nation. But medicine now played a large part. Doctors were more readily available to all classes of society. Hospitals no longer existed for the care of the sick but for the treatment of illness. Surgery was rapidly becoming a curative science. Prevention of some diseases was now possible and, above all, the cause of many had been discovered. In 1800 medicine was still an empiric art. In 1900 medicine possessed a scientific basis.

At the beginning of the nineteenth century the doctor's main function was the alleviation of symptoms. He possessed a large armamentarium of drugs, some of which are still in use today. The pharmacopoeia was a mixture of ancient and modern. A *Clinical Guide*, popular among Edinburgh students in 1801, lists useful remedies like castor oil, opium and digitalis but still contains such alchemic potions as syrup of pale roses, crabs' eyes, pearls and the 'sacred elixir'. Thus the practitioner could treat constipation, relieve pain and steady the pulse. But he could only rarely deal with the underlying cause of his patient's illness for the simple reason that the cause of most diseases was as yet unknown. Possessing few aids to diagnosis, he must depend upon his senses, sight, hearing, touch, smell, even taste. There is a story of a well-known physician summoned in consultation by a practitioner who found himself baffled by a mysterious fever. 'Typhus' said the physician as they came to the sickroom door. 'But you haven't even seen my patient' protested the doctor. 'No. I've smelt him,' answered the physician. 'Typhus fever always smells of mice.'

The early nineteenth-century medical man prided himself upon his detailed knowledge of gross anatomy. To him the body was a single entity, made up of easily identifiable structures arranged in an orderly relation: the nerves, veins, arteries, muscles, bones, heart, lungs and stomach. Disease only affected organs and structures: the bladder, uterus, kidneys, cartilage or skin. A diseased organ could often be detected in life by surface inspection or deep palpation. After death the diagnosis could be confirmed by autopsy, provided the disease process was visible to the naked eye.

Marie Francois Xavier Bichat, a surgeon in the French Revolutionary Army, was the first to break away from this concept of organs. In 1799—1803 he formulated and published a theory of tissues or membranes, suggesting that every body structure is made up of components and that disease does not necessarily affect the whole organ but only one of the tissues of which it is composed. Bichat fell into error, attributing fixed properties to each of his twenty-one varieties of tissue and classifying them like chemical elements. His ideas formed the basis of work done by Jean Cruvelhier at Paris in 1836—42. Cruvelhier advanced the theory that a disease process is always due to a morbid secretion into the tissues of an organ. Again this is an error, but one which had the effect of inducing Carl Rokitansky of Vienna to enquire more closely into the structure of organs. He performed over 30,000 autopsies himself and examined an equal number of specimens sent by other workers. Rokitansky published several beautifully illustrated books between 1839 and 1875, in which he described a number of important discoveries, throwing new light on diseases of the lungs, liver and kidneys and on congenital defects of the heart. Rokitansky has some claim to be regarded as the founder of modern pathology.

All the findings of Bichat and Cruvelhier depended upon naked-eye appearances. So did most of Rokitansky's work. The microscope played little part in medicine until the middle of the nineteenth century. Instruments of a kind had been in use for a very long time but were not sufficiently powerful to reveal organisms smaller than amoebae and the very largest bacteria. The arrangement of lenses blurred the object under examination, because they were placed haphazardly in the tube and the reflected light rays from the mirror divided into a spectrum. The brothers Chevalier first attempted to remedy this defect in 1823. In 1830 Joseph Jackson Lister, father of the more famous Joseph Lister, produced a truly achromatic instrument by using doublets, a plano-concave lens of flint glass cemented to a convex lens of crown glass. Freed from chromatic distortion and spherical aberration, the microscope became capable of revealing particles far beyond the range of unaided vision. It is strange that J. J. Lister's essential modification has gone largely unnoticed, except in specialist journals, yet his son's whole work depended upon an efficient miscroscope.

In 1831 Mathias Jacob Schleiden, a German professor of botany, observed the cell nucleus by means of the microscope. Shortly afterwards Theodor Schwann, an anatomist and physiologist, discovered nucleated cells in animal tissue. Schleiden and Schwann met by chance at a dinner party and discussed their findings. As a result of this conversation, Schwann began a deliberate search of every tissue known to him. In 1839 he wrote a book upon his work, in which he enunciated the theory, regarded as the most important generalization in the science of morphology, that the structure of animal and vegetable tissue is essentially similar. 'There is one universal principle of development for the elementary parts of organisms, however different, and that principle is the formation of the cells.' Schwann, a devout Catholic, feared that his cell-theory might be regarded as heresy and submitted his manuscript to the Bishop of Malines. This should remind us that religious doctrine still exerted a profound effect on science in the nineteenth century. An even more striking example is to be found in the bitter controversy aroused by the later theories of Darwin and Pasteur.

A German professor, Jacob Henle, applied Schwann's work to medicine. In 1841 he wrote the first treatise on microscopical histology, classifying tissues and dealing with their development and functions. In 1866—71 he published epoch-making volumes describing a number of discoveries in the microscopical anatomy of the brain and nervous system, muscles, viscera and blood vessels. Another of his works is *A Handbook of Rational Pathology*, really a new type of medical text book, in which he laid down that all disease is a deviation from normal physiology and that the physician should therefore be able to anticipate or prevent disease as well as attempting to cure it. Another German, Albert von Kölliker, went a little further than Henle by applying Schwann's cell theory to embryology, showing that the ovum is a single cell and that the organism's growth depends solely upon cell division.

All these investigations and theories, although important in themselves, may be regarded as preliminary to the momentous work of Rudolf Virchow, professor of pathological anatomy at Würzburg and Berlin. In his hands the cell theory became the basis of modern medicine. Virchow published his *Cellular-Pathologie* in 1858. He postulated that the body is a 'cell-state in which every cell is a citizen'. The cells, he wrote, could not grow independently but derived one from another. Thus a tumour is not an entirely new growth of cells, but is always formed from pre-existing cells. The process of disease causes normal cells to become distorted or to proliferate at an abnormal speed.

Virchow's teaching radically altered previous concepts both of disease and of the human body. No longer could the body be seen as a single entity or a simple collection of tissues, the different parts clearly visible to the unaided eye and demonstrable by gross dissection. The new concept saw the body as a mass of cells, each one endowed with individual life and capable of undergoing change. A disease process might be shown by the changes in these cells, rendered visible by the microscope. Thus the cell theory opened up an entirely new field for research. If the disease process depended upon abnormal behaviour of normal cells, then the cause of disease could be found in the reason why cells behave abnormally. The answer or answers to that question have not yet been fully worked out. But Virchow's cell theory had another effect. The practising doctor began to lean heavily upon the laboratory pathologist. The pathologist required an efficient microscope, some method of staining specimens so that cell envelopes and nuclei could be clearly differentiated, and a means of cutting thin sections to obviate blurring. The first suitable stain, a mixture of carmine, ammonia and gelatin, was introduced in 1847 by Joseph von Gerlach of Mainz, and this was the stain used by Virchow himself. The thin sections were at first cut by hand with a razor. In 1866 Wilhelm His introduced the microtome, but the instrument did not come into common use until 1875. The microscope increasingly became a diagnostic aid from the middle of the nineteenth century. As yet it did not reveal the cause of disease but helped to establish the site and nature.

In 1835 Charles Cagniard-Latour examined yeasts under the microscope and found them to be composed of small globules, apparently of a living, vegetable kind. Two years later Theodor Schwann confirmed his findings and showed that the 'yeast plant' causes fermentation which can be suppressed by heating. At that time the science of chemistry was dominated by Justus von Liebig, who had established a teaching laboratory at Giessen in Germany. Liebig, a pure materialist, refused to believe that fermentation was anything but a chemical process or that yeasts could be endowed with life. It is recorded that he obstinately refused even to examine yeasts under the microscope. The majority of scientists inclined to Liebig's view that fermentation was a simple inorganic chemical reaction.

About 1857 Louis Pasteur, professor of chemistry at the University of Lille, started to investigate the nature of ferments. He examined lactic acid fermentation of milk, alcoholic fermentation of wines and beers, butyric fermentation which turns butter rancid, and acetic fermentation which makes vinegar. He showed that each process depended upon a specific ferment, i.e. there exists a milk-souring ferment and an alcohol-forming ferment and the two are not interchangeable in action. Continuing his experiments with milk, Pasteur concluded that the responsible ferment was living and capable of reproduction. He found that ferments needed warmth for proliferation but were killed by too high a temperature. Then he discovered the important fact that if he heated the fluid and securely sealed the containing vessel, milk would remain unfermented for an apparently indefinite period.

Since airtight sealing seemed essential to the preservation of milk from fermentation, Pasteur turned his attention to the part played by air. Souring, putrefaction and infection had always been held to have much in common. General opinion maintained that all three were caused by bad air or miasma. Pasteur was not satisfied with this explanation. He had already observed microscopic yeasts and other microorganisms. He had noted that yeasts proliferate by division. There seemed to be only one source for extraneous ferments which caused so much trouble to vintners by souring their wine. The obvious source was the surrounding air. Putting these facts together, Pasteur concluded that air was not itself to blame but a ferment carried by the air. He prepared glass tubes, filled them with milk, blood or urine, drew the tube ends out to a fine capillary, and bent the capillaries at an angle. He then submitted the tubes to a degree of heat sufficient to destroy any ferment present in the fluid. Pasteur found that no putrefaction or fermentation occurred. Yet the fluid was in contact with air. The fine bore of his capillaries and the stagnant column of air contained in the bend did not permit entry of microorganisms.

Thus Pasteur was led to his Germ Theory. He unfortunately over-dramatized his findings when describing his experiments to the Sorbonne University on 7 April 1864. Telling of a flask of milk which he had sterilized and kept airtight for some months, he declared:

And I wait, I watch, I question it, begging it to recommence for me the beautiful spectacle of the first creation. But it is dumb, dumb since these experiments were begun several years ago; it is dumb because I have kept from it the only thing Man cannot produce, from the germs which float in the air, from Life, for Life is a Germ and a Germ is Life.

The exact meaning of this well-known passage is not clear. Pasteur seems to imply that his 'germs' are the cause of life, that without the vitalizing germ all matter is dead. Such was the meaning read into his statement at the time. But Pasteur had quite probably been carried away by his own exuberance and had intended to imply only that the living process of fermentation could not proceed in the absence of the essential organism. He had already become embroiled in a controversy as to the origin of life, which revolved around the spontaneous generation of 'germs'. A vessel containing sterilized fluid sometimes 'went bad'. Did the organisms of putrefaction develop spontaneously in the fluid or had they entered from outside through a fault in the seal? Pasteur had clearly shown the latter to be the case when he made his tubes with bent capillaries—in fact this was the whole point of his experiment. He performed these experiments before 1861, yet his statement of 1864 was not clear and could be translated into a claim that he had discovered the cause of life itself.

The controversy split the medical profession—and not the medical profession only—into two fiercely contending factions. Pasteur's discovery of 'germs' came at a critical time, when confidence in the age-old concept of created Man had been shaken by the publication of Charles Darwin's *On the Origin of Species by Means of Natural Selection* in 1859. His *Descent of Man* (1871) struck an even greater blow at fundamental teaching. Man was no longer the centre of the Universe, created by an all-wise God to exercise dominion over everything upon earth. He had reached his dominant position by a process of natural selection. All plants and animals, including Man, had developed from less complex beings and would continue the process of development. The theory of evolution was not new, but the proofs put forward by Darwin and his application of the theory to Man were revolutionary. Darwin cast doubt upon the story of the Creation as related in the first chapter of Genesis. There were many who held that Pasteur's 'Germ of Life' disproved the existence of a Creator.

It is difficult for us now to understand the fierce passion aroused. Certainly never in the history of medicine, and probably never in science, has a controversy lasted for so long a time and been so bitterly argued. The new theories seemed to strike at the very roots of accepted belief. There were many wise, earnest and thoughtful men who found themselves genuinely unable to accept evidence incompatible with religious doctrine. There were others who saw a new scientific age, free from superstition, dependent on fact and not upon faith. There were many more who tried to correlate the new discoveries with ancient tradition, and these produced some fascinating theories though they are now forgotten. The controversy had two major effects, one bad, one good. It was harmful because it induced unscrupulous opposition to those who put Pasteur's discoveries to practical use and so retarded the advance of medicine, and particularly surgery, for over ten years. It was good because of the wide and intense interest aroused. The bulk of the medical profession were made acutely aware that something revolutionary might have been found and eagerly awaited convincing proof or disproof.

On 3 August 1864 Thomas Spencer Wells, a surgeon at the Samaritan Hospital, London, addressed the annual meeting of the British Medical Association at Cambridge. Wells told of some recent advances made in the field of medicine and he mentioned Pasteur's work:

> Applying the knowledge for which we are indebted to Pasteur of the presence in the atmosphere of organic germs which will grow, develope, and multiply, under favourable conditions, it is easy to understand that some germs find their most appropriate nutriment in the secretions from wounds, or pus, and that they so modify it as to convert it into a poison when absorbed—or that the germs after development, multiplication, and death, may form a putrid infecting matter—or that they may enter the blood and develope themselves, effecting in the process deadly changes in the circulating fluid.

Here is fairly clearly stated the potential importance of Pasteur's Germ Theory to medicine. But Wells also indicated the difficulty. Did germs 'after development, multiplication, and death . . . form a putrid infecting matter' or did 'they enter the blood and develope themselves, effecting in the process deadly changes in the circulating fluid'? In other words, are germs simply a product of disease or do they cause disease?

No one could give the answer. Many bacteria had been seen by 1864, revealed under the microscope as rods, chains or spherical bodies. They undoubtedly occurred in various diseases, but it seemed impossible to prove their exact function in the disease process. The point was argued for over ten years. In 1876 Robert Koch, a general practitioner in the district of Wollstein, Germany, started to investigate the problem. He had no special training and no elaborate laboratory, but had for some time been interested in microscopy and spent much of his spare time examining specimens. In April 1876 Koch reported to a botanist, Ferdinand Cohn of Breslau, that he had made a special study of the anthrax bacillus, which is common in horses and cattle and can be transmitted to man. Koch did not discover the large anthrax bacillus, which had been seen many times before and was accurately described by Franz Pollender as early as 1849. But Koch succeeded in isolating the bacillus and growing it in a culture medium. Cohn invited him to continue his experiments in the Breslau laboratory, where Koch made a number of discoveries. He found that, given warmth and oxygen, the bacilli formed spores in the blood and tissues of animals. The spores were able to survive in the absence of warmth and oxygen to develop into bacilli when conditions were again favourable. Thus the soil might become infected with anthrax spores and produce the disease if they entered the tissues of a warm-blooded animal. Cohn published Koch's findings later in 1876.

There now occurred one of those strange incidents, very common in the annals of science, when two or more people pursue a similar line of research, quite unaware that anyone else is working on the subject. Koch probably studied anthrax because he lived in an agricultural district and farmers were mystified by outbreaks occurring in fields from which cattle had been excluded for many years. French agronomists believed the disease to be caused by an inorganic poison. Early in 1877 Louis Pasteur, then unaware of Koch's work, decided on an investigation. He had already produced pure cultures of yeasts and other ferments by growing them in suitable media. He now found by experiment that anthrax bacilli rapidly multiplied in urine, and he seeded 50 cc of sterilized urine with one drop of blood from an infected animal. He allowed the culture to grow and then seeded a second 50 cc of urine with one drop of the culture. Proceeding in the same manner, he produced a dilution of the original drop approximately to 1 in 1,000 million. The blood was not now perceptible, but the culture teemed with anthrax bacilli because they had multiplied throughout the sub-cultures. Pasteur found that one drop of his end product, when injected into a healthy warm-blooded animal, caused death from anthrax just as certainly as did one drop of blood from an infected animal. He had proved that the disease anthrax must be attributed to infection by the anthrax bacillus.

Pasteur, satisfied that his 'germs' were the cause and not a product of disease, now tended to concentrate his investigations on the attenuation of their virulence, work which has been briefly mentioned in Chapter 5. Robert Koch continued to investigate the methods of reproduction and habits of microorganisms. He was greatly helped by the introduction of aniline dyes, used as stains to show up bacteria in microscopical preparations. In 1878 he identified six different types of bacteria which caused surgical infections, and he proved that each of the six bred true through several generations. Three years later, in 1881, he succeeded in producing pure cultures (they had previously been more or less contaminated with other organisms) by transplanting selected colonies from generations grown on glass plates covered with a nutrient medium of gelatine and meat infusion. This is the forerunner of the well-known 'Petri dish' introduced by Koch's assistant Julius Petri in 1887. Koch was thus able both to grow and to inoculate pure cultures of various disease organisms. In 1882 he described his best-known discovery, the tubercle bacillus, and in the same paper laid down the rules governing the relationship between bacteria and disease:

1. The organism must be found constantly in every case of the disease.
2. It must be possible to cultivate the organism outside the body of the host in pure cultures for several generations.
3. The organism, isolated and cultured through several generations, must be capable of reproducing the original disease in susceptible animals.

These are Koch's Postulates and, when they are applicable, prove conclusively that a specific disease is caused by a specific organism.

It had now been shown that bacteria cause a number of diseases. The fact obviously changed the theory and practice of medicine during the late nineteenth century. Diagnosis, prevention and, in due course, cure all became more simple and more certain. While every branch of medicine was more or less affected, the Germ Theory produced its first and most dramatic results in surgery. Operative surgery had been almost entirely destructive until the end of the eighteenth century, undertaken only when all other attempts at cure or alleviation failed. Unbearable pain, crippling deformity, or imminent death were the indications for operation. Surgeons sometimes attempted constructive repair but the agony and high mortality did not justify such experiments. Operating speed was the criterion of a good surgeon. He had little time to think out his next step or to consider the best means of dealing with an unexpected difficulty.

Half-hearted attempts to allay the pain of surgery have been made from time immemorial. There was nothing in the nature of a deliberate search and the methods used were ineffectual.* It needed an alteration in

---

* The Ancients possessed two agents, opium and alcohol, which are pain-allaying drugs. Opium would have been ineffective as an anaesthetic unless used in dangerously large doses. Physicians tended to regard alcohol as a stimulant and therefore did not permit the surgeon to administer alcohol

Footnote continued on p. 142

the public attitude towards suffering and increasing ambition of the surgeon before the pain of surgery would become a problem to be urgently tackled. The necessary combination developed during the first four decades of the nineteenth century. Men such as Astley Cooper, Aston Key, Robert Liston, James Syme and William Fergusson advanced operative surgery far beyond the simple amputations and lithotomies of tradition but found their full capacity limited by the pain which they unavoidably inflicted. A more humane pattern of behaviour became apparent. In the 1830s Dr Thomas Arnold of Rugby did much to suppress the bullying, profligacy and indiscipline which disgraced public schools under such 'flogging headmasters' as Keate of Eton and Boyer of Christ's Hospital. An Act of 1833 abolished slavery throughout the British Empire. In the same year Lord Althorp's Factory Act set limits to the hours worked by children. Lord Shaftesbury's Mines Act of 1842 prohibited employment of women and children underground. The prize ring was driven into hiding by 1837 and officers taking part in or promoting duels were liable to be cashiered by an amendment to the Articles of War in 1844. Reforms in service discipline and of the penal code and the institution of a civil police force in 1829 are all indications of a more humane and ordered way of life. The introduction of anaesthesia in 1846 is not a casual discovery but a dramatic outward expression of an inner and very real change from eighteenth century brutality to our own more tender attitude towards suffering.

Humphry Davy can be credited with the first suggestion of a practical means of anaesthesia. In 1800 he wrote 'As nitrous oxide in its extensive operation appears capable of destroying physical pain, it may probably be used with advantage during surgical operations in which no great effusion of blood takes place.' Little attention was paid to his suggestion, although his book on nitrous oxide received lengthy and favourable reviews. The gas was used successfully by Horace Wells, a dentist of Hartford, Connecticut, in 1844 but proved unreliable. Sulphuric ether had been known for many years and entered the pharmacopoeia as an 'antispasmodic' for the treatment of asthma and croup. Sniffing or drinking of impure ether, as a substitute for alcohol, became prevalent especially in Ireland and America. The first administration of ether for surgery, by Crawford Long of Jefferson, Georgia, on 30 March 1842 resulted from these 'ether frolics'. Long was himself an addict and the same is probably true of his patient, James Venables. The incident had no effect upon the successful introduction of anaesthesia, not having been reported until several years after Morton's experiment.

William Thomas Greene Morton, a dentist who had been in partnership with Horace Wells, deliberately used ether as a substitute for nitrous

---

Footnote continued from p. 141

except for that purpose. When the surgeon worked single-handed, for instance in the Navy or in rural America, he often made the patient drunk before operation.

oxide. The question of whether he approached the subject in a scientific spirit is controversial and still in dispute. Morton is known to have administered ether to a patient named Eben Frost for the extraction of teeth on 30 September 1846. Two weeks later, on Friday, 14 October 1846, he gave a public demonstration in the operating theatre of the Massachusetts General Hospital. The senior surgeon, John Collins Warren, removed a small tumour, probably a tuberculous gland, from the neck of Gilbert Abbott, a twenty-three-year-old house painter. The entirely successful demonstration took three minutes. Those three minutes changed the whole craft of surgery.

The news spread round the world with remarkable speed. It has been said that, within a year, hardly an operation was performed without the aid of ether. Opposition was trivial, a sure sign that anaesthesia had been introduced at the psychologically correct moment. But ether suffered from several disadvantages and was soon replaced by chloroform, introduced by James Young Simpson of Edinburgh in 1847. Simpson, an obstetrician, used chloroform for the relief of pain in labour. Obstetric anaesthesia aroused much opposition. The opponents were of the male sex and usually clergymen. They based their objection on two common fallacies. First, it is natural for a mother to suffer when bearing a child and relief of pain will lessen maternal affection. Second, the curse laid upon Eve is 'in sorrow shalt thou bring forth children'. The first objection is still occasionally made today. The second reminds us that the literal interpretation of Holy Writ (as laid down in the Authorized Version) was a valid argument in the 1840s. Simpson fought his opponents by every means in his power but he made little headway until 1853 when, at the command of the Prince Consort, John Snow administered chloroform to Queen Victoria at the birth of her eighth child, Prince Leopold. Thereafter obstetric analgesia became known as *'chloroform à la reine'* and opposition gradually died down. Here is a striking example of how Royal approval can set a fashion not only in attire but in matters of greater public interest.

Anaesthesia conferred two benefits upon surgery. It not only freed the patient from pain but gave the surgeon *time*. The second resulted from the first and is the greater gift. No longer limited by the urgent demand for speed, a surgeon was able to perfect his techniques and to embark upon procedures hitherto impossible. Surgery became constructive. Repairs of hernias, excision and reconstruction of diseased joints in place of amputation, were now undertaken. The number of open operations greatly increased. In 1846 a surgical ward of thirty beds might contain eight operation cases at any one time. The remaining twenty-two were patients suffering from illness or accidents not requiring operation or judged unsuitable for surgery. In 1860 the respective figures would have been twenty-five and five.

But open operation—that is a 'cutting' operation, one in which the protective skin is broken—carried a grave risk. Wounds became infected, leaked pus, and took a long time to heal. All too frequently a more severe infection developed, became generalized, and resulted in death. It is often said that anaesthesia actually increased the risk by rendering surgery possible. In fact, this is not entirely true. The total mortality of surgical wards, due to all causes, varied only fractionally at around 12 per cent in 1846 and 1860. The operative death rate actually fell from 11.8 per cent in 1846 to 9 per cent in 1860. Since five times the previous number of patients underwent operation, and 9 per cent of operative cases died, the total number of deaths was much higher than before the introduction of anaesthesia. About 66 per cent of these deaths were due to 'hospital disease', that is to generalized sepsis.

Surgeons recognized the danger and made valiant attempts to combat sepsis. The classical picture of the callous surgeon in his blood- and pus-stained frock coat, tying ligatures with his teeth, and snuffing 'the good old surgical stink' like a warhorse scenting battle is little better than a myth. They used a number of drugs and methods. The drugs were classed as 'antiseptics' which meant what the name implies, a medicament alleged to combat developed sepsis, and all were ineffectual. In the middle years of the nineteenth century, surgeons turned increasingly to attempted prevention by means of a 'kitchen-clean' technique which depended upon irrigation with quantities of cold boiled water. Thomas Spencer Wells, the first British surgeon to understand the importance of Pasteur's Germ Theory, strongly advocated the technique and saw no good reason to alter his method because of germs. He was a specialist in the very dangerous procedure of ovariotomy, the only abdominal operation then commonly undertaken. In 1864, despite strict adherence to 'cleanliness and cold water', 33 per cent of his ovariotomy patients died and his colleagues regarded this as a low mortality.

Joseph Lister apparently did not read Wells' address to the British Medical Association. He first heard of Pasteur's work through a chance conversation with Thomas Anderson, professor of chemistry at Glasgow University. Lister must have been one of the very few surgeons of his time able to accept Pasteur's findings without question. His father, J. J. Lister, a wine merchant, was a self-taught natural scientist particularly interested in the microscope. A Quaker, he regarded instruction of his children as more desirable than frivolous amusement. Thus Joseph Lister was familiar with the problems of fermentation and had been conditioned to accept the existence of organisms outside the range of unaided vision. Pasteur's Germ Theory came to Lister not so much as a revelation but as a simple explanation of a problem with which he had long been familiar.

Pasteur's germs probably caused surgical sepsis, but how could they be prevented from entering a wound or attacked once they had invaded the tissues? Lister turned to crude carbolic or German creosote which in 1863 had been suggested as a wound dressing by Jules Lemaire of Paris. The sequence of events is not clear but Lister probably made an unsuccessful trial of carbolic as an 'antiseptic' in March 1865, before he had heard of Pasteur's theory. By August he had decided that a scab, Nature's own wound dressing, if impregnated with carbolic would form a barrier to Pasteur's germs and might kill those that had already invaded the surface tissues. He used this method on 12 August 1865 when an eleven-year-old boy, James Greenlees, was admitted to Lister's male accident ward at the Glasgow Royal Infirmary. Greenlees had sustained a very dangerous injury, a compound fracture of the tibia. Compound fractures were particularly dangerous because the open wound, with much damage to tissues and bone, formed an easy path for infection. Lister covered the injury with carbolic-impregnated lint and laid sheet metal over the lint. The lint, soaked in blood and serum, formed an artificial scab. Simple removal of the metal plate allowed fresh carbolic to be painted over the surface of the lint and so to form a barrier through which microorganisms could not pass.

Greenlees' leg healed without trouble. On 16 May 1867 Lister published the results of his treatment in eleven cases of compound fracture. Eight had made uneventful recoveries. Two had been attacked by hospital disease. Both recovered, one after amputation of the limb, one after conservative treatment. One patient died, but death was caused by the broken bone-end piercing an artery and was not due to sepsis. Eight uneventful recoveries in a series of eleven compound fractures, with only one death, was a record of success never before attained in this type of injury.

Lister now started to develop a technique suitable for elective operations. In common with many others, he fell into Pasteur's error that pathological organisms were entirely carried by the air. After experimenting with various methods, he devised in 1872 a steam-powered carbolic spray, capable of filling a large room with carbolized mist. Reason dictated that the operation site should be at the centre of this cloud, and Lister ensured that the spray thoroughly soaked his hands and instruments. It followed that the spray erected an efficient antiseptic barrier, although the theory underlying its use was incorrect. Lister, by ensuring that no living bacteria could pass the barrier, produced an *aseptic* operating field by means of a chemical *antiseptic*. This important fact is too often not recognized.

The majority of surgeons did not at first appreciate the principle underlying Lister's method and regarded it as 'the carbolic treatment' which might or might not prove superior to other techniques. Opposition to Lister rapidly developed when it became apparent that his teaching depended upon acceptance of the Germ Theory. Contrary to opinions expressed in many popular biographies of Lister, opposition was not confined to London and was no more intense in London than in other centres. Lister had fierce opponents and equally ardent supporters among surgeons in every city and in every country. He received particularly strong support in Germany, where army surgeons had tried his method with good results in the Franco-Prussian War of 1870, and this is the reason why the immense forward thrust of surgery in the last quarter of the nineteenth century was pioneered by the Germans. Lister's operating theatre and wards at Edinburgh, to which he moved from Glasgow at the end of 1869, became thronged with visitors from all over Europe, including London.

Many surgeons simply waited. They required undoubted proof that

Lister's technique was an advance before they abandoned their own methods. Lister, after one disastrous essay in statistics, refused to publish any more figures. The *Lancet* vainly pleaded that a surgical ward in a London hospital should be set aside for a full and unbiased trial. In 1877, twelve years after his first use of carbolized lint, Lister accepted the vacant chair of clinical surgery at King's College, London, with an associated surgeoncy at King's College Hospital. He came to London in October and the chance of proving the superiority of his method occurred within less than a month.

Francis Smith, a forty-year-old billposter, sustained a simple fracture of his right patella on 12 October 1877 and was admitted to Lister's ward. Lister attempted to unite the two fragments by traction but failed to secure union and announced his intention of incising the skin and wiring the fractured bone together. The proposed operation broke one of the strictest rules of old-fashioned surgery. A simple fracture might cause disability if it failed to unite, but carried no risk to life or limb. Compound fractures carried so high a mortality that immediate amputation was generally advocated. Lister, by incising the protective skin, would turn a simple into a compound fracture. Many surgeons held that he proposed wantonly to risk his patient's life for the sake of a quite unjustifiable experiment. On Friday, 26 October, Lister cut down on the fracture and wired the two fragments together. Francis Smith walked out of King's College Hospital on 11 January 1878. By modern standards the operation was trivial but here was the long awaited proof that Lister's technique could enlarge the bounds of surgery.

Sir John Erichsen, senior surgeon to University College Hospital, remarked in 1874 'The brain, the thorax and the abdomen will forever remain closed to the hands of the wise and humane surgeon.' Every one of these areas had been explored before 1900. Not only did the scope of surgery widen, but the danger of operation lessened. Lister, in the years 1877–93, achieved the very low operative mortality of 1.5 per cent but his work was almost, although not quite, confined to a type of operation which would now be described as minor orthopaedic and accident surgery. His more ambitious assistant, W. W. Cheyne, experienced an operative mortality of just under 3.5 per cent in the same period, and the figure is generally accepted as approximately correct for late nineteenth century surgery. Lister's technique reduced operative mortality by 66 per cent and these much better results were obtained by the virtual elimination of generalized sepsis which had caused two-thirds of deaths before.

Carbolic is a dangerous antiseptic. Surgeons and scientists strove to find a safer but equally effective substitute. Bacteriological examination revealed that the vast majority of air-borne microorganisms are harmless. In 1883 Elie Metchnikoff discovered the existence of phagocytes, cells in the bloodstream capable of destroying the few pathogenic organisms which might be expected to enter an operation wound from uncontaminated air. German surgeons recognized that dirty hands, instruments and dressings are the most potent source of infection. Instruments could easily be sterilized by heat. Steam sterilization began to be applied to all articles used in an operation. There followed sterilized gloves to cover hands which cannot be rendered surgically clean, caps to prevent contamination from the hair, face-masks to inhibit droplet infection. The spray was found to be unnecessary and carbolic increasingly went out of use. By 1900 many surgeons had switched from an 'antiseptic' to an 'aseptic' technique. The First World War, fought in a highly manured terrain and producing the gross damage of high explosive, showed that antiseptic drugs, being protoplasmic poisons, delay the healing of injured tissue. Since they can only destroy bacteria by direct contact, they proved not only useless but actively dangerous in the treatment of wounds massively and deeply infected. At the end of the war, only a very few old-guard 'Listerians' clung to antisepsis. The great majority had adopted asepsis. Hardly one surgeon understood that the two methods were similar in principle and differed only in practice.

Meanwhile chemists were searching for the perfect antiseptic, one which would be effective against pathogenic bacteria but harmless to the body tissues. In 1906 Elie Metchnikoff published his theory that soured milk is an intestinal antiseptic, a substance which can be swallowed without harm yet will destroy hurtful microorganisms in the intestinal tract. His theory stimulated the search. Having produced no less than 605 useless preparations, Paul Ehrlich and S. Hata synthesized their 'magic bullet', an arsenical drug originally thought to be effective against a wide range of bacteria. The famous salvarsan or 606 proved lethal only against the Treponema group, of which *Treponema pallida*, the spirochaete of syphilis, is the best known. Salvarsan and its successor neosalvarsan are examples of the 'perfect antiseptic' because they were capable of curing syphilis by direct action upon the causative organism without inflicting gross disturbance of the body functions. Salvarsan was the only known means of *curing* an acute infection until the time of the Second World War. Although *Pasteurella pestis*, the cause of bubonic plague, was discovered in 1894, a person suffering from plague could not have been cured. Had a great epidemic occurred in Western Europe at any time before 1939, physicians would have been as helpless to *cure* their patients as were doctors in the Black Death. They could only have assisted the patient's own resistance to the infection.

Experience gained in the First World War suggested that certain dyestuffs, flavine for example, are fairly efficient antiseptics and relatively harmless. In 1935 a German chemist, Gerhard Domagk, discovered that a derivative of the dye chrysoidin, prontosil rubrum, cured mice infected with streptococci. Prontosil R was marketed as a systemic antiseptic but later in 1935 three French workers found that the complex dyestuff contained a simpler and already known constituent, sulphanilamide. From this developed the group of 'sulfa drugs'. May and Baker 693 or sulphapyridine, successfully used from 1938 in the treatment of pneumonia, is perhaps the best known. Sulfa drugs are not true antiseptics but rather bacteristatics which keep the organism in a state of enfeebled existence and so assist the normal body mechanism in its struggle to overcome the invader.

In 1876 Professor John Tyndall reported that the thick, felty growth of a mould *Penicillium glaucum* caused the death of bacteria grown in mutton broth. He thought death to be caused by simple deprivation of oxygen. A similar observation was made by others, including Joseph Lister. One year later Louis Pasteur and Jules Joubert found that the large anthrax bacillus is sometimes destroyed by smaller organisms. This led Pasteur to suggest that one organism might deliberately be set to make war upon another. He was applying the principle of antibiosis, the old idea that one species exists at the expense of others, e.g. that a tiger preys upon the deer which preys upon grass. In 1928 Alexander Fleming observed this phenomenon when a culture of staphylococci became accidentally contaminated by a penicillium mould. Fleming prepared a crude broth extract and found it lethal to a quite large range of pathogenic organisms when injected into rabbits. He also found his penicillium broth to be no more toxic to the animal than an injection of plain broth. He reported his findings, gave the name 'penicillin' to his broth filtrate, but attempted no clinical trials. His work was taken up by Howard Walter Florey and Ernst Boris Chain at the Sir William Dunn School of Pathology, Oxford, in 1939. Two years later they were manufacturing a crude penicillin, first used clinically by C. M. Fletcher at the Radcliffe Infirmary in 1941. With American help, a sufficient supply for limited use had been built up by 1943. In 1958 more than 440 *tons* of pure crystallized penicillin was produced by America alone.

Penicillin destroys organisms and so *cures* infections. It kills by interfering with the nutrition of the organism and bacteria can resist this interference. Since bacteria increase by division, resistance will be conferred upon the progeny. Thus a penicillin-resistant strain of bacteria will develop. Despite this great disadvantage, which can be a real danger if antibiotic drugs are misused, penicillin and its successors have proved their undoubted value in the cure of infections.

Many other major advances in medicine date from the nineteenth century. Among them is one of the greatest of diagnostic aids, X-rays or, as they should be properly called, Röntgen rays. In November 1895 Wilhelm Konrad Röntgen, professor of physics at Würzburg, was investigating cathode rays by means of a Crookes' tube when he noticed that curious shadows were being cast by various objects in his laboratory. He surrounded the Crookes' tube with a close fitting shield of black paper, thereby cutting out a possible source of light, and found that the shadows were thrown by objects in front of a platino-barium screen, standing nine feet away, which itself shone with a greenish fluorescent glow. The strangest point was the variation in intensity of the shadows. Some things appeared quite black against the glowing screen while others, although not translucent in ordinary light, appeared only faintly outlined and threw no shadow at all. Röntgen described his discovery in the *Proceedings* of the Würzburg Physico-Medical Society on 28 December. A translation, by

Arthur Stanton, appeared in the British scientific journal *Nature* on 23 January 1896.

So far as is known, the first diagnostic use of Röntgen rays was at Liverpool. On 22 February 1896 the *Lancet* described the localization and subsequent removal of an air gun pellet in a boy's wrist. The surgeon concerned was Robert Jones, the famous pioneer of orthopaedic centres and accident services, while the photographs were taken by the even more famous Oliver Lodge, then professor of physics at Liverpool. Realization that X-rays are not only an essential diagnostic aid but also a means of treatment led to the work of Pierre and Marie Curie on radioactivity and their isolation of a radium salt in 1902. There is little doubt that Marie Curie thought that she had discovered 'the cure for cancer' and the hope was shared by many others. Results did not prove good, but the discovery of radium led to the use of radioactive emanations through the radon seed or 'gold grain' to the radium, cobalt and caesium 'bombs' which have been very successful in the treatment of certain types of cancer.

The science of genetics, which later threw new light on the nature of some diseases, had its beginnings in the mid-nineteenth century. The story is so well known as to need only brief mention. Gregor Mendel, a Roman Catholic monk, experimented with the growing of various types of peas in the abbey garden of Brunn in Austria. He discovered that when tall peas were crossed with short peas, the progeny followed a regular pattern. He postulated that a true tall pea contained two elements of tallness, a true short pea two elements of shortness, and that only one of each element would be transmitted to the progeny when crossed. Mendel also observed the phenomenon of dominance, when he found that a true tall crossed with a true short will always be tall, and that shortness will appear only in a quarter of the next generation.

After ten years of experiment, Mendel published his theory in 1866. It attracted no attention and remained buried in the pages of an obscure journal for thirty years. Then three botanists in three different countries had the same idea. During their researches they found that Mendel had done similar work and that his conclusions were correct. In 1905 William Bateson, working on the hybridization of sweet peas at Cambridge, gave to Mendel's hereditary factors or elements the name of 'genes'.

Genetic mutation is now believed to be the reason why living organisms of all kinds are capable of adapting themselves to varied conditions of life, that is evolution depends upon continuing changes in the hereditary genes. The question of whether it is permissible to assist mutation so as to breed out undesirable characteristics and breed in desirable ones is controversial and is commanding attention at the present time. Genetics can be considered as an area of critical examination. X-rays were a dramatic advance, a discovery certainly deserving the modern term 'a breakthrough'. The same is true of anaesthesia and the discovery of radium. All these, and many other lesser nineteenth-century findings, added up to produce a revolution in medical thinking and practice. But the fundamental difference between eighteenth-century medicine and that of the twentieth is to be found in two entirely new concepts. First, in the concept of body structure as a cell-state, composed of individual cells and developing from a more primitive organism. Second, in the evidence that bacteria, equally endowed with the attributes of development and generation, not only exist but are capable of causing disease. This is why the 'cell theory' and the 'germ theory' must be accorded the first place in changing medicine from an empirical art into a science.

9 Towards a National Health Service

The medical discoveries and the social reforms of the nineteenth century could not have benefited a sufferer from disease unless accompanied by equally great advances in the care of the sick. There were marked improvements in accommodation, treatment, nursing and diet. Let us start with a very necessary development, a change in the attitude towards mental illness. Until almost the end of the eighteenth century madness was universally regarded as akin to crime, a very old idea expressed in the phrase 'possession by the devil'. In the few hospitals which catered for the insane, such as the famous St Mary of Bethlehem or Bedlam, lunatics were confined to cells and loaded with chains. Restraint was the only recognized form of treatment. In France in 1793, at the height of the Terror, Philippe Pinel of the Bicêtre Hospital in Paris asked permission of the Paris Commune to free selected lunatics from their bonds. The time was inauspicious because Robespierre and others of his colleagues in the Committee of Public Security already suspected that wanted aristocrats were being hidden in the Paris hospitals. The Commune reluctantly gave permission for the experiment, more on the grounds that Liberty demanded freedom from chains than in the belief that they were helping to advance medical science. Pinel found his life endangered, partly because of the suspicion that he was helping aristocrats to escape, partly because of popular fear that numbers of homicidal maniacs would invade the streets. In fact, only one lunatic made a bid for freedom and he was easily persuaded to return. Pinel discontinued this first experiment but he received permission for a renewed trial from the National Assembly on 24 May 1798. He freed forty-nine patients from their chains and found their condition to improve rapidly when no longer forcibly restrained. In 1801 he published a book describing his methods and this exerted a profound effect on the treatment of lunacy.

In 1791 a Quaker patient died as the result of cruel treatment at the York County Asylum or Madhouse. William Tuke, a Quaker philanthropist and merchant, suggested to the Society of Friends that they should found their own institution where mentally afflicted Friends might be cared for in a more humane fashion. This famous asylum, The Retreat at York, opened in 1796 with accommodation for thirty patients. Tuke was not a physician and had not heard of Pinel's experiments. He is usually given credit as the first man to institute humane treatment of lunatics in Britain but there is reason to believe that he followed the example of a less well remembered Quaker, Dr Edward Long Fox.

Fox, a Bristol physician, had a particular interest in mental illness. He was a republican and is known to have visited Paris on several occasions during the years following the Revolution. He probably met Philippe Pinel in 1793. In the following year, 1794, Fox took charge of a small private asylum at Cleeve Hill on the outskirts of Bristol. This seems to have already belonged to the Society of Friends. In 1795 Fox publicly announced that he had enlarged the house, and there is no mention of any restriction to members of the Society. Four years later he decided on a much greater expansion and purchased an estate for the purpose at Brislington, on the main road between Bath and Bristol. Here he built an asylum on an entirely new plan, which opened in 1804 to house seventy patients. The asylum admitted both paying and non-paying lunatics. Every patient had a separate room opening on to a court in which were kept tame silver pheasants and doves. Fox encouraged his patients to look after these birds, and whenever their condition permitted, he gave them suitable employment in the house and grounds. He would allow no one to stay in bed unless physically ill. Common rooms and entertainments of various kinds were provided, but he insisted on rigid segregation of the sexes. Even in the chapel, served by visiting clergy of all denominations, women sat on one side and men on the other.

Active treatment largely depended on hypnosis. Suggestion has been part of medical treatment from time immemorial. 'Stroking' was popularized for a time in the seventeenth century by Valentine Greatrakes who claimed the ability to stroke pain away. This stroking movement became known as magnetism and formed part of the technique used by Franz Anton Mesmer, an Austrian Swiss who enjoyed enormous success in Paris during the decade before the Revolution. An aura of charlatanry has always surrounded mesmerism, although it is the basis of psychoanalysis. Fox practised mesmerism extensively under the older name 'animal magnetism'. There is a well authenticated story that he tamed a bull by this method, on which he rode round Bristol to visit his patients and so to demonstrate the usefulness of animal magnetism. He was also a pioneer in the treatment of madness by 'balneology', using various forms of bath at Brislington, and buying houses and the island of Knightstone at Weston-super-Mare as a seabathing station for his patients. Although an eccentric man (like his great friend Thomas Beddoes of Bristol) Fox became the most successful and best known alienist of his day. In 1811 he was commanded to Windsor in consultation with the royal physicians, who suggested that he might be asked to take charge of George III. Fox declined the offer probably because of his strongly republican views.

In 1807 a select committee of the House of Commons recommended the establishment of public asylums for the maintenance of pauper and criminal lunatics, implemented by the 'Wynn Act', 1808, but little action resulted. Another scandal at the York Asylum in 1814 instigated the setting up of a committee to visit and report upon all madhouses in England. It is interesting that the committee reported very favourably on the management of Brislington House, but this was exceptional. The great majority of establishments, including Bethlehem, were filthy, under the charge of cruel and ignorant keepers. Another select committee in 1827 closely investigated conditions in Middlesex; the report of this committee instigated foundation of the Middlesex County Pauper Lunatic Asylum at Hanwell in 1831. In 1839 John Conolly was appointed medical officer to this, the largest mental hospital in Britain, and at once abolished all forms of mechanical restraint. Conolly based his work on that of Pinel and disseminated the idea of non-restraint through his writings. By 1845, when local justices were compelled to provide asylums chargeable to the poor rate, the concept of restraint had given place to the concept of seclusion.

'It must be remembered that we are an asylum rather than a hospital' wrote C. H. Cottrell, chairman of Colney Hatch, in his report to the select committee on lunatics in 1859. The large county asylums formed enclosed communities, their inmates supported from parish rates and employed according to their abilities in workshop and farm. The doctors in charge were alienists, physicians who looked after people excluded from ordinary life. They could not yet call themselves psychiatrists, practitioners who specialized in the treatment of the human mind. The theory that disease is a divine affliction was no longer credited. Nineteenth century discoveries in science and medicine tended to suggest that *all* disease is somatic or physical. Physicians now looked for a physical cause. Since there must be a cause for mental aberration, they searched the patient's past history to uncover the explanation. They divided causes into 'moral' and 'physical', moral if insanity could be attributed to a precipitating incident, physical if the patient was already physically ill when insanity developed. Among physical causes were intemperance, masturbation, over-study, injury and severe illness. Moral causes were legion, ranging from shocks, marital difficulties and domestic grief to such oddities as sudden loss of several cows and over-excitement at the 1851 Great Exhibition. If the physician could uncover no definite reason, he made the diagnosis of 'hysteria', signs and symptoms not indicative of a disease process but manufactured by the patient. The term 'hysteria' derives from the Greek word for 'womb' and therefore has a sexual connotation. For this reason many doctors preferred 'hypochondria' when the subject was male.

Study of hysteria is the starting point of psychiatry and depends largely upon the work of Charcot and Freud. Jean Martin Charcot of the Saltpêtrière Hospital in Paris was certainly not the first to recognize the existence of nervous disease but he did more than anyone to differentiate somatic 'neurology' from animist 'psychology'. Sigmund Freud worked with Charcot in 1885 and accepted his finding that hysteria is not necessarily connected with sex. Hysteria is amenable to cure by suggestion and Freud therefore studied hypnotism. His findings led Freud to divide the brain into three levels, conscious, pre-conscious and sub-conscious. The subject could not recall experience stored in the lowest level unless assisted by the hypnotist or psychologist. Assistance could be given not only by hypnosis but also by allowing the patient to talk at random. A skilled psychologist might then be able to follow an association of ideas which led him to the underlying reason hidden in the sub-conscious. Thus Freud developed the method of psychoanalysis which is, in essence, the release of repressed experience from the sub-conscious into the conscious mind, enabling underlying trouble to be rationally explained. Although much of Freud's teaching has met with opposition, his methods form the basis of modern psychiatry and have revolutionized the treatment of mental disorders.

Care of the sick was generally unsatisfactory at the beginning of the nineteenth century. The urge to found hospitals died away at a time when rapidly increasing town population demanded more beds. Such hospitals as existed were 'voluntary', depending upon voluntary subscriptions and medical attendance. Admission to a voluntary hospital could usually only be obtained by presentation of an order from a subscriber or governor. The system tended to be abused in an age when any middle class family employed a number of domestic servants. Too many governors regarded their subscriptions as a convenient means of freeing themselves and friends from the responsibility for the care of sick dependants. In 1827 William Marsden found a girl lying almost on the point of death in Bedford Row. Enquiry revealed that the sick woman had been turned away by more than one hospital because she could produce no 'letter' and that no subscriber whom she had approached would give her one. Marsden opened a Dispensary for the Sick Poor to which any needy person might apply. His dispensary developed into the Royal Free Hospital, the word 'Free' denoting that no letter of recommendation was required.

Hospital nursing had deteriorated to a low level, though not so low as is suggested by the familiar figure of Mrs Gamp. Many nurses cared for their patients to the best of their ability and with considerable acquired skill. But all were untrained and generally lacked even rudimentary education. Nurses belonged to the servant class and, when employed in private houses, were regarded as equals of the scullery maid rather than of the upper servants. They probably drank no more and were no more immoral than other women of the same social status but the drunkard and the lecher had greater opportunity in hospitals than in well conducted households. The prevailing medical fashion for a 'supporting regimen' made large supplies of alcohol available in the wards and the presence of a number of young apprentices and house pupils encouraged prostitution.

The need for reform had been recognized in the 1820s when a London physician, Dr Gooch, unsuccessfully tried to introduce some kind of disciplinary training. In 1833 Pastor Theodor Fliedner of Kaiserswerth in Prussia, assisted by his wife Friederike, turned his garden house into a refuge for discharged female prisoners and in 1836 started a school of Lutheran deaconesses which rapidly developed into a large Order mainly concerned with the care of the sick. Mrs Elizabeth Fry visited Kaiserswerth in 1840 and founded her Institute of Nurses on returning to England. She achieved only a limited success. A few London hospitals accepted her probationers as assistant nurses but, so far as can now be ascertained, Mrs Fry removed them after they had gained some experience and employed them in private nursing.

Hospital wards were not attractive to women of any refinement. The occupants, filthily dirty and teeming with vermin, suffered from many diseases only rarely seen in England today: delirium tremens, typhus fever, and the last stages of pulmonary tuberculosis are examples. The stink of illness and of surgical infection in particular nauseated all but the most hardened. Even medical students found themselves revolted by the combination of dirt, drunkenness, immorality, pain and despair. Many teachers used unnecessarily frank language and coarse behaviour before their pupils with the object of inuring a sensitive lad to hospital life. A situation had arisen in which no respectable woman would consider nursing the wards while such conditions prevailed yet reform was impossible until respectable women could be induced to undertake the work.

The legend that this reform was accomplished by Miss Florence Nightingale is so widely accepted that there is little real hope of altering the traditional story. Yet Miss Nightingale would have been the first to deny the truth of the legend. She believed the independent Sisterhood to be the best method of nursing a hospital and she regarded the now forgotten Sister Mary Jones as the woman who had done more than any other to reform hospital nursing. Her *Notes on Hospitals* and her letters to Sister Mary make both points clear. Reform was initiated by the Anglican Nursing Sisterhoods, of which St John's House or the Sisterhood of St John the Evangelist was the first and most influential. Founded in 1848 largely through the interest of Robert Bentley Todd, an eminent physician on the staff of King's College Hospital, St John's undertook full responsibility for nursing the hospital on 31 March 1856. In the following year, 1857, Sister Mary Jones started a training school through which all her probationers must pass before being accepted as nurses of St John's House. Under her charge, the order and decency of the wards became notable. Delegations from all over Europe studied her nursing methods throughout the next decade. The Russian Orthodox Nursing Sisterhoods, which did excellent work until the 1917 revolution, are said to have been instigated by a report of the delegation sent to King's College Hospital by Tsar Alexander II. By 1866 St John's nursed the two London teaching hospitals of King's and Charing Cross besides a hospital at Nottingham, the Leicester Infirmary, and the well known English or Galignani Hospital in Paris.

In 1859 the Trustees of the Nightingale Fund, a sum of money subscribed as some tribute to her work in the Crimean War, urged Miss Nightingale to decide how the fund should be used. They suggested a large extension of training at St John's House. Sister Mary had by now become one of Miss Nightingale's warmest friends but the proposal proved unworkable because only members of the Church of England could be accepted at St John's. After an abortive approach to the London Hospital and after discarding a scheme for an entirely new institution, Miss Nightingale decided to found her school of nursing in conjunction with St Thomas' Hospital where the Matron, Mrs Wardroper, had the reputation of one of the best in London. Miss Nightingale was doubtful of success for St Thomas' at that time occupied temporary premises, the medical staff suspected the plan, and few probationers of good quality could be recruited. The Nightingale School at St Thomas' opened on 24 June 1860 with fifteen pupils.

In these early years, the two schools had differing purposes. St Thomas' existed, in Miss Nightingale's own words 'to train training matrons'. That is, a graduate was expected to head an untrained staff and to train it to Nightingale perfection. The St John's school at King's existed to train nurses. As Miss Nightingale and Sister Mary cooperated closely together, there was much interchange between the two schools, St John's Sisters going to St Thomas' for a time for training as 'matrons', Nightingale trainees attending St John's to study their methods of training nurses. A typical example is Miss Burt, who founded the famous Guy's Hospital training school in 1879. She had attended the Nightingale School and, as a Sister of St John's House, had been Sister-in-Charge of the Leicester Infirmary.

This close cooperation and the intimate friendship of Miss Nightingale with Sister Mary combined to produce the District Nurse. District nurses, first on their bicycles and later in their Baby Austins, became a familiar feature of the English countryside and played a no lesser part in the towns. 'The Nurse' implied to the poorer class a District Nurse rather than her colleague in a hospital. Generations of poor people depended upon her for skilled care in their own homes. The first was a woman sent to St John's House in October 1857 by Lady John Scott for training as a visiting nurse 'in the extensive village of Cawston [near Rugby] and its neighbourhood'. The Council of St John's decided that this was a very proper use for their institution; by 1859 a number of women had been trained for the purpose and the time had come to consider an extension of their usefulness.

Miss Nightingale had interested herself in the experiment from the beginning. She now joined Sister Mary in urging that midwifery training should be added to experience gained in medical and surgical wards. Both ladies were of the opinion that a single-handed nurse without a midwife's experience was almost valueless. The St John's Council, Miss Nightingale and Sister Mary now joined in bringing pressure to bear on King's College Hospital. Most hospitals strongly objected to lying-in wards because one case of puerperal fever would usually infect all patients. Students learned their midwifery 'on the district', that is by attending women in their own homes. The hospital rather unwillingly agreed to make a ten-bedded ward available for the sole purpose of training women, temporarily attached to St John's House, as visiting or 'parish' nurses. 'The Nightingale Ward' opened on 7 January 1862, the cost of equipment and maintenance being borne by the Nightingale Fund. For the next six years applicants to both the St John's school and the Nightingale school were divided into two batches, those judged more suitable for hospital nursing being sent to St Thomas', those better suited to the special conditions of district nursing being sent to King's.

In 1859 Mr William Rathbone, a philanthropic ship-owner of Liverpool, employed one nurse to tend patients in a Liverpool slum. Finding one nurse to be hopelessly inadequate, Rathbone determined to employ more, but they necessarily had to be of a trustworthy type and such women were hard to find. The story of what now happened is not clear, but Rathbone seems to have prepared plans for a school rather similar to that at King's and sent his plans for Sister Mary's approval on 27 June 1860. Sister Mary did not altogether approve and raised her objections in a letter to Miss Nightingale dated 29 June. These documents only came to light in 1974, having been stored in the archives of the Community of St Mary and St John, founded by Sister Mary when she seceded from St John's House in 1868. In the following year, 1861, Rathbone came to London to discuss his proposals with Miss Nightingale and Sister Mary. By their advice, he opened at his own expense a school for District Nurses associated with the Liverpool Royal Infirmary in 1862.

The nursing of 1885 differed greatly from that of 1848 but now the Nursing Sisterhoods were rapidly losing support and influence. There are two reasons for this decline. The first was common to both Miss Nightingale's trainees and the Sisterhoods. In the early days, control of a nursing staff could only be entrusted to a 'lady', an educated woman usually wealthy and of some social standing. All too often these condescended to their work, regarded themselves as 'gifted' to clear up the mess made by the ignorant male, and treated their colleagues, administrators and medical staff alike, as underlings whose sole duty lay in obeying their commands. Miss Nightingale experienced endless trouble of this kind. The fact is that her trainees had considerably less nursing skill and hospital experience than the nurses whom they came to train, a disability which resulted in unwise rules and continual friction. The trouble became less acute when trained nurses began to take the place of 'ladies' as heads of the nursing staff, but it persisted for many years. The Sisterhoods did not survive as influential bodies into this less troubled era. Many, but no means all, of the Sisters exacerbated the conflict by allowing their religious exercises to take precedence over the welfare of patients under their care.

The second reason for the decline of the Sisterhoods is their unwavering attachment to the High Church. At first welcomed as self-denying women, prepared to give their lives to the care of the sick, they soon came under attack as proselytizers, determined to drag patient and nurse alike to the feet of the Pope. Their behaviour was not calculated to allay suspicion. Let us admit that. (A book on the history of medicine is not the place to discuss the rights and wrongs of the case. The author must be allowed to express his opinion, without arguing the evidence, that the hypocritical and often fraudulent charges made against these devoted and useful women by protestant bigots form a deplorable chapter in the history of the Church of England.) The Sisterhoods were defeated by propaganda and this is one reason why they are now almost forgotten. It is indeed fortunate that they retained influence until such time as the non-sectarian nursing schools, founded by hospital management committees on the lines of Miss Nightingale's, were sufficiently well established to take over the work.

Voluntary hospitals were hopelessly insufficient in number to cater for the needs of the sick. We have mentioned that Parliament failed to implement the full proposals made by Edwin Chadwick (p. 101). He had never evisaged that aged and sick should be accommodated in his repressive workhouses. Some attempts were made to alleviate sick paupers by outdoor relief and the attendance of parish doctors, but most Boards of Guardians found it cheaper and more convenient to admit them to the workhouse. In 1834 about 10,000 workhouse inmates needed medical care and the number had risen to over 50,000 in 1861. Pressure on voluntary hospital beds increased the problem. Voluntary hospitals became selective in the type of case admitted. By 1861 the majority of 'general' hospitals would not admit children, the chronic sick, or patients suffering from epilepsy, mental disorders, syphilis, advanced tuberculosis and skin diseases. The Fever Hospital, Islington, and two workhouses were the only London institutions willing to accept patients suffering from infectious disease. Very few specialized hospitals existed, except for the lying-in hospitals which were not desirable because of the great risk of puerperal fever. Small children's hospitals opened at Liverpool in 1851, Great Ormond Street, London, 1852, Norwich and Manchester in 1853. Another specialized institution, the Royal Hospital for Incurables, Putney, dates from 1854. In 1861, when the population of England and Wales stood at just over 20 million, 117 hospitals with under 12,000 beds provided the only accommodation for persons in need of hospital treatment.

About the year 1862 William Rathbone became distressed by the kind of treatment given to pauper patients at the Brownlow Hill Institution, part of the large Liverpool Union. The Institution had the reputation of being unusually well managed and was at least separated from the workhouse. Rathbone found conditions to be dreadful and particularly criticized the nursing, performed by able-bodied paupers under the direction of untrained parish officers. He asked Miss Nightingale to supply a Matron and nurses, offering to pay the cost himself. Miss Nightingale sent a party of twelve Nightingale nurses, headed by Miss Agnes Jones—no relation of Sister Mary. The party took charge of the male wards on 16 May 1865.

They found the wards unspeakably disgusting, far worse than in any London voluntary hospital. Miss Jones intended to train pauper-nurses as assistants, but they proved hopeless. The Master had favoured a new system but found himself faced by a furious Miss Jones, who roundly blamed him for all deficiencies and demanded that he carry out her orders. The Board of Guardians backed their Master, technically the superior of the Matron. It seemed as though the experiment must fail but Miss Nightingale intervened and persuaded Miss Jones to be more tactful. The strained atmosphere gradually relaxed and the nurses more than proved their worth. The doctors recognized their merits, asked for more trained nurses, demanded that the female wards be also placed under their charge. Miss Jones, an able administrator, actually managed to reduce the cost of maintaining the infirmary despite all her improvements. She worked herself to death, never going to bed before 1.30 am, rising again at 5.30. Early in 1868 the crowded wards were visited by typhus fever. Agnes Jones caught the infection. She was a woman of magnificent physique and indomitable will but had overtired herself and died on 19 February 1868.

Her success and her martyrdom paved the way for general reform of the workhouse and its infirmary—or so it seemed. The reformers encountered apathy and opposition. A number of public spirited people, ably assisted by Miss Nightingale from her couch in South Street, formed various societies dedicated to the cause. In 1865 James Wakley, owner of the *Lancet*, had been prompted by a number of workhouse doctors to make an investigation. He commissioned three London physicians as inspectors. They produced an admirable report, drawing attention to a number of faults, but the document is of outstanding interest because it contains the sentence 'The state hospitals are in the workhouse wards.' This is the first occasion on which anything in the nature of a State Hospital Service had been acknowledged to exist.

As complaints poured in and public concern mounted, the Government decided on action. Mr Charles Villiers, President of the Poor Law Board, prepared to introduce a Bill, largely drafted by Miss Nightingale, but the Government fell before he had the opportunity. Others were working behind the scenes and, on 8 February 1867, the new President, Mr Gathorne Hardy, introduced his Metropolitan Poor Bill. Hardy had omitted to consult Miss Nightingale, who angrily tried to arouse opposition. During the long debate it became apparent that the Bill had too many merits for any party to oppose it seriously. The Bill aimed to remove all children, lunatics and fever patients from workhouses, made provision for the erection and improvement of infirmary buildings, and instituted payment of staff from a general rate and not by the parish in which the workhouse stood. The Act applied only to the metropolitan area, but is generally regarded as the first step towards a National Health Service.

Next year the Poor Law Amendment Act empowered provincial authorities to provide separate infirmaries. Even in the 1860s building cost money and progress was slow. All but three of the thirty Metropolitan Poor Law areas had separate infirmaries before 1883, but very few had been built in the provinces. A census of sick poor taken as late as 1896 showed that of 58,550 sick only 22,100 were in separate infirmaries, the large remainder being tended in general workhouses. Exactly half the infirmary patients were in twenty-seven metropolitan institutions. These separate infirmaries were, on the whole, well equipped and well run. By 1888 all London infirmaries had been put under the charge of a medical superintendent. Formerly the parish doctor had been subordinate to a lay Master, often ignorant and dictatorial. The superintendents, many of whom had already worked as house officers in voluntary hospitals, not only supported their junior staff against oppressive local authorities but strove to raise the standard of patient care to voluntary hospital level. Since superintendents possessed the medical knowledge which Guardians lacked, Boards found themselves no longer able to argue on equal terms, as had been the case with their lay Masters, and were forced to grant the requests of their medical superintendents.

Throughout the late nineteenth and early twentieth centuries, the worst aspect of the infirmaries was the quality of their nursing. This is strange when we remember that introduction of a Nightingale staff to Liverpool started the movement for reform. An acute nursing shortage developed between 1880 and 1900, partly due to the decline of the Sisterhoods and partly to the difficulties experienced by voluntary hospitals in maintaining adequate recruitment to their own training schools. Success of Low Church agitation came at a particularly unfortunate time for infirmary nursing. In 1885 no Board of Guardians could possibly have considered employing a High Church Sisterhood in the wards of their infirmary. Yet this is just the type of work which the Sisterhoods would have eagerly undertaken. Boards of Guardians did their best but many reported that all patients were tended by trained nurses when, in fact, one trained nurse supervised the efforts of completely untrained paupers. Conditions gradually improved as the voluntary hospital schools enlarged and as the infirmaries started to train their own staffs and to provide better pay and living conditions.

The 1867 Act created a new body, the Metropolitan Asylums Board which also had the duty of providing London with fever hospitals. The Board achieved a certain success, although some of the accommodation provided in obsolete battleships and an aged cross-Channel steamer was not exactly first class. Greater knowledge of epidemiology suggested the advisability of isolating all patients who suffered from infectious disease. In the smallpox epidemics of 1871 and 1876, investigation showed that about 80 per cent of patients in the London fever hospitals were not paupers but in gainful employment. This led to a prolonged and complicated parliamentary wrangle because the facilities had been provided under the Poor Law. In 1889 the Metropolitan Asylums Board was empowered to admit non-paupers, that is paying patients, and so became the hospital authority for all cases of infectious disease in London. Two years later, magistrates were empowered to order detention of fever cases in hospital and, at the same time, charges for accommodation were abolished. The practice gradually extended over the whole country. The Third Reform Act of 1884 extended Household Suffrage to all classes but still debarred inmates of Poor Law institutions. The Act produced a quite extraordinary anomaly. An impoverished patient in a voluntary hospital was not a pauper and therefore allowed a vote. A well-paid artisan who happened to be suffering from an infectious disease might be automatically disenfranchized because he temporarily inhabited one of the Poor Law fever hospitals. The Medical Relief Disqualification Removal Act of 1885 remedied this absurd situation by permitting the sick pauper to vote. Thus, by 1891, every inhabitant of London and of many provincial towns had become entitled to free hospital treatment without stigma of pauperism or electoral disqualification. The principle of a State Hospital Service had been established.

Let us now turn to the kind of medical treatment available for the worker who did not need a hospital. The domiciliary service provided under the Poor Law was unsatisfactory. District medical officers employed by Boards of Guardians were usually part-time and of a low standard because the post offered no attractions either in pay or nature of work. Except in country districts, where he was the sole practitioner available, the 'parish doctor' attended only the most poverty-stricken class. The great majority of wage-earners depended upon the 'sixpenny doctor', often an able but over-worked general practitioner who received patients in his surgery, gave them a cursory examination, and invariably supplied a bottle of more or less harmless medicine, bright colour and pungent flavour being the most desirable qualities. He also signed the certificate enabling his patient to draw sick pay. Other sources of medical advice were the free dispensaries, generally very well run, and the outpatient departments of voluntary hospitals, which usually required a 'doctor's letter' of recommendation.

Sick pay came from the clubs or mutual benefit societies which had started to develop at the end of the eighteenth century. These were financed by regular weekly payments of a small subscription from their members. Benevolent gentry usually managed the club in a country district but in industrial areas the club was democratically administered by its own elected committee. Fraudulent conversion of funds became rather common and many of the smaller clubs failed through the defalcation of a dishonest treasurer. Many others were well run and some coalesced into nationwide societies of a quasi-masonic type bearing names such as Oddfellows, Foresters, Druids, and the Ancient Order of Buffaloes. The clubs not only provided sick pay but sometimes employed their own doctors. The larger clubs not infrequently founded cottage hospitals, capital and part of maintenance being provided by employers. Although excellent in intention, the club system suffered in practice from the dis-advantage of any voluntary scheme. Benefit only accrued to the provident who would, by some means or other, have saved for emergencies. The improvident, who had no thought except to spend money as soon as earned, must rely upon parish doctor and relieving officer.

Dissatisfaction with the Poor Laws led to the setting up of yet another Royal Commission in 1905, which reported in 1909. Their findings are of little importance when compared to the minority report signed by Mrs Beatrice Webb, Mr George Lansbury and Prebendary H. Russell Wakefield. These urged a state medical service on the lines of the compulsory insurance scheme which had been introduced by Bismarck and had operated in Germany since 1883. The signatories stressed that the imperfections of administering the Poor Law were totally irrelevant. They called into question the official attitude towards poverty. It should be recognized that poverty was no crime, but a consequence of defective social and economic organization. Thus, care of the sick poor should be the responsibility of the 'state', that is of the whole community.

Two minor breaches in the Bastille of the Poor Laws had already been made by the Unemployed Workmen Act of 1905 and the Old Age Pension Act of 1908. When the Chancellor of the Exchequer, David Lloyd George, introduced the latter measure, he implied that pensions would in time become part of a compulsory insurance scheme. During his Budget speech in the following year he again mentioned national insurance. Despite these warnings, his introduction of the National Health Insurance Bill in 1911 came like a thunderclap. The volatile little Welshman had been remarkably tactless, omitting to consult interested bodies and discarding practically every recommendation of the 1905 commission. This is the reason why Lloyd George's Bill evoked such violent opposition, not least from those whom it would most benefit. Workers strongly objected to any deduction from wages and were not impressed by the famous slogan 'ninepence for fourpence', the contribution of worker, employer and exchequer. Lloyd George insisted upon free choice of doctor, thus infuriating those like Mrs Beatrice Webb who demanded a benevolent 'state' dictation. Club doctors feared loss of income. They did not accept Lloyd George's calculation that the average club doctor received an annual payment of 4s. to 4s. 6d. per patient, whereas the Insurance Commissioners would pay a capitation fee of 7s. 6d. Lloyd George stood firm despite intense opposition and secured passage of his Bill. The National Health Insurance Act was appointed to come into force on 15 July 1912.

The medical profession as a whole mildly welcomed the Act. Dr J. Smith-Whitaker, one of the first Insurance Commissioners to be appointed, had served as Medical Secretary of the British Medical Association since 1902, and his appointment aroused no protest. General practitioners formed the backbone of the scheme and it became necessary to negotiate the detailed implementation of the Act with their representatives. The most convenient representative body was the BMA. It seems that the Council of the BMA genuinely did not appreciate that *national* health insurance must imply some degree of national, that is government, control. Only when negotiations started did the Council understand that doctors must accept a measure of subordination to the Insurance Commissioners. Relations between the negotiating bodies became strained. The BMA advised their members not to work under the Act. Meetings of the Association branches throughout the country gave the impression that doctors were unanimous in opposition. The BMA required its members to sign an undertaking that they would refuse to serve until the government accepted almost impossible conditions put forward by their Council. So fierce did opposition seem that the Act was not enforced on the appointed day.

'Professional unanimity' applied only to the top. Club doctors and sixpenny doctors were by no means satisfied with existing conditions. They could expect a better rate of pay under the insurance scheme and, so oppressive was the rule of many clubs, that their doctors did not fear the bogey of 'government interference'. Resignations from the BMA increased every month during the second half of 1912. Early in January 1913 David Lloyd George, unmoved by all the excitement, announced that he had enlisted nearly 10,000 doctors willing to accept service and capable of attending almost 14 million insured persons. The BMA had no option but to release its members from their pledges. The 'great panel war' ended in a somewhat undignified scramble for patients. The National Insurance Act, applying to about 15 million workers, came into full operation by the end of 1913.

The Act provided a free general practitioner service and sickness benefit paid through approved societies, such as trade unions and large clubs. Local insurance committees could also distribute benefit to dependants of insured persons requiring sanatorium treatment but, in general, only the insured worker could obtain free advice and treatment. Medical research received a subsidy of $1d$. per insured person per annum, the money being administered by the Medical Research Committee, which became the Medical Research Council in 1920.

The Act suffered from grave defects. It applied only to wage-earners who received an income of less than £160 a year, and did not affect civil servants or teachers in this bracket. Payment through approved societies led to great differences in the amount of sickness benefit. Drafts of the Bill had never been referred to any committee of experts in local administration, public health, medical practice, or even insurance. Lloyd George did not consult the Local Government Board. In consequence local authorities played no part and these could probably have administered the service far more ably, economically and fairly than the cumbersome insurance committees and approved societies. The worst feature resulted from Lloyd George's abysmal ignorance of medicine and his failure to consult the profession. The Act gave the worker free consultation with his doctor and financial assistance but did nothing to improve his treatment in illness. The old club and sixpenny practitioner persisted under the new name of panel doctor, his primary purpose still to sign the certificate and provide the magic bottle of medicine. Framers of the Act did not grasp the essential fact that the hospital is the prerequisite of sick care when the patient is unable to afford skilled diagnosis and domiciliary nursing. The panel doctor could deal only with trivial illness, minor injury and some chronic disease. The acutely ill or seriously injured worker must still depend upon voluntary hospital and infirmary.

The white-collar class of worker could obtain no form of hospital treatment before 1880. They were in the unfortunate position of being too wealthy to merit admission to voluntary hospitals, too proud to enter an infirmary, and too poor to afford expensive home nursing. Henry Burdett, a stockbroker who had served as secretary to Queen's Hospital

Birmingham, drew attention to the miserable plight of sick lodgers and produced a scheme for the foundation of 'Home Hospitals' in 1877. A small pay-hospital opened in Northampton in 1879 and the Hospital for Women, Soho Square, made a wing available for paying patients in the same year. On 27 June 1880 the first of Burdett's Home Hospitals opened in Fitzroy Square, London, and proved immediately popular. Joseph Lister made frequent use of this home. The voluntary hospitals found it difficult to make ends meet and favoured Burdett's scheme. The new St Thomas' proved much too large to be maintained out of available resources. At one time the Governors could afford to open only thirteen of the twenty-one wards. Burdett's Home Hospital Association proposed to use the empty blocks for paying patients. The suggestion aroused opposition, but was implemented as the St Thomas' Home for Paying Patients on 1 March 1881. The home provided two single rooms at four guineas a week and a large number of cubicles at 56s. In 1884 Guy's Hospital, financially crippled by lack of support following 'the great nursing dispute', opened a small number of pay-cubicles and at the same time started to charge one guinea a week for accommodation in the ordinary wards, patients in real need being admitted freely as before. This system of payment spread rapidly to other hospitals. By 1890 15 per cent of provincial hospital income came from this source. Many of the provincial infirmaries made a charge for accommodation whenever practicable.

Church collections had raised money for the upkeep of hospitals since the early eighteenth century. In 1873 the rather unorganized effort became consolidated into the Hospital Sunday Fund. The Saturday Fund, administered by working men's clubs, followed in 1874. During the 1880s workmen subscribing to the Fund started to claim the *right* to hospital treatment in return for their weekly pennies. In 1895 the Hospital Almoner Service began work with the appointment of Miss Mary Stewart at the Royal Free. Almoners not only sought to relieve hardship but also tried to ensure that patients able to afford payment did not abuse the free treatment available. In 1903 members of the Saturday Fund complained to the governors of St George's Hospital, London, that the almoner had no right to apply a 'means test'. There were quite ugly scenes in the board-rooms of hospitals at Belfast and Swansea when a number of workers invaded meetings of the governors and demanded free treatment, without interrogation, in return for their subscriptions of 1d. a week.

During the last two decades of the nineteenth century a number of nursing homes, quasi-charitable institutions and small specialist hospitals had come into operation. Many were well run and served a useful purpose. Many were little better than sleazy lodging houses. A few were blatantly fraudulent. It was too easy for a medically qualified rogue to found a 'hospital' for the treatment of a particular disease, attract subscriptions by advertisement, and charge his patients high fees. The secretary of one quite reputable hospital for diseases of the skin allocated to himself 15 per cent of all receipts from patients' payments and charitable donations.

Infirmaries were not only increasing in number but offering amenities approaching those of the voluntary hospitals. Ratepayers failed to see why they should be required to support these 'palatial workhouse infirmaries' and also be pestered for money by the voluntary hospitals. The latter fell into still greater financial difficulty. Some, Guy's for instance, began to charge for outpatient attendance, a move which angered public and general practitioners alike.

In 1889 dissatisfaction prompted an enquiry undertaken by the House of Lords. The investigation applied only to London hospitals. The Lords committee issued a report in 1892, their chief recommendation being that all London hospitals should be placed under control of an independent central board of forty-nine members. The report ended with a warning that all hospitals would find it necessary to seek government or municipal support unless urgent action was taken. Argument took the place of action, while the large voluntary hospitals fell rapidly and more deeply into debt. In 1896 Henry Burdett and Alfred Fripp, a young surgeon on the staff of Guy's Hospital, enlisted the interest of the Prince of Wales. The Prince invited a number of leading doctors, financiers, industrialists and Church dignitaries to meet him and discuss the critical hospital finances. This powerful group agreed to collect and administer a fund, the interest to be distributed by a general committee. The Prince of Wales' Hospital Fund for London to Commemorate the Sixtieth Year of the Queen's Reign raised over £800,000 before the end of 1902. Investigation showed that part of the hospitals' financial trouble resulted from amateur methods of costing and accountancy. The Fund committee therefore decided that no hospital should receive benefit unless it adopted a standard method of accounting. In the first four years the Fund paid for the reopening of 433 beds, closed because of financial stringency. A number of small hospitals were persuaded to amalgamate into more economically viable units. By 1910 the Fund provided about one-tenth of the total monies required by the London voluntary hospitals for annual maintenance. King Edward's Hospital Fund for London, as it was renamed, fulfilled the main functions of the central board proposed by the House of Lords. It was never sufficiently powerful nor did it ever possess a large enough income to ensure an efficient hospital service but, without the Fund, the situation would have ended in disaster.

The First World War accustomed all classes to the idea of hospital treatment for serious injury. Down-the-line clearance of casualties from the trenches to the base hospital in England suggested that the same kind of scheme might be applied to civilian patients. In 1917 David Lloyd George, now Prime Minister, set up a Committee which became the Ministry of Reconstruction under Sir Donald Maclean. The Maclean Report advised abolition of Boards of Guardians and transfer of their functions to county and borough councils. This entailed transfer of infirmaries, but the Report made no recommendations regarding voluntary hospitals. Lord Rhondda, President of the Local Government Board, favoured a scheme putting both Poor Law infirmaries and voluntary hospitals under government control, with free medical attendance for all and no element of charity. Two more or less unofficial committees worked on the problem. The first, under the aegis of Mrs Webb and members of the Labour party, assumed the creation of a Ministry of Health and that the Minister would be responsible for a National Health Service. The second, headed by Major Bernard Dawson, later Lord Dawson of Penn, also visualized a Ministry of Health and a Service. The plans produced by these committees were surprisingly similar. Both insisted on the integration of preventive with curative medicine. The Labour plan introduced the term 'health centre', avoided for the present by Dawson. The BMA feared the Labour plan would entail a government-controlled and salaried service. Sidney Webb reassured them that the scheme allowed for private practice. The BMA replied that the views of the Labour party closely agreed with those of their Council on the subject.

Lloyd George's coalition government was returned to power on 7 December 1918. His election manifesto promised that care and treatment of the sick should cease to be administered under the Poor Laws but become part of a general health service. The Ministry of Health was set up in 1919 to fulfil the election promise, the first Minister being Dr Christopher Addison, a qualified medical practitioner. Addison immediately appointed a Council on Medical and Administrative Services, under the chairmanship of Sir Bernard Dawson. The Council never issued a final report. As the proposed reorganization was presumed to be a matter of urgency, they published a preliminary report for discussion in 1920. This revolutionary plan is one of the more important, although tragic, documents in the history of British medicine.

Dawson's Council considered existing medical services insufficiently well organized to bring the advantages of medical knowledge or the advances recently made in treatment within reach of all people. The interim report laid particular emphasis on the need to bring preventive and curative medicine together. Here the general practitioner must be the meeting point. His duties should embrace not only medicine as applied to the individual but as applied to the community. Infant welfare, prenatal care, school clinics must all form part of the general practitioner service. The 'family doctor' should have at his command laboratory accommodation, dental surgeries and recuperative facilities—which presumably meant convalescent homes. This greatly extended scope of a GP's work necessarily implied some degree of cooperation and a large increase in surgery premises and equipment. Dawson therefore now accepted the Labour proposal for Health Centres. But he introduced an element of RAMC wartime organization. The Primary Health Centre would resemble a Casualty Clearing Station, staffed by general practitioners having a limited number of beds under their care, possessing sufficient laboratory facilities for everyday needs, and suitable for clinical examinations of the type required in preventive medicine. Consultant advice would be available at the Primary Health Centre, but the main working area of consultants and specialists would be in the Secondary Health Centre, located in a hospital capable of undertaking diagnosis, care and treatment of the more difficult case. Dawson thought that such a scheme must inevitably bring general practitioner and consultant more closely together with consequent benefit to both.

The Council did not favour a full-time salaried service which they thought might discourage initiative and encourage mediocrity, but accepted the payment of both general practitioners and consultants on a part-time basis. They did not agree on the question of fee-paying patients in the service. Some members upheld the principle of free service for all, but the majority objected on the grounds that a large number of people could afford at least part of the cost of treatment and total dependence on Exchequer or local authority would impose too severe a burden on public funds. The scheme would cost a great deal of money. The Council considered that most cottage hospitals and some infirmaries could be adapted as Health Centres, but rebuilding would be necessary on a large scale. Since the report was an interim one for discussion, there were a number of important omissions. The Council gave no exact details of administration and, perhaps purposely, they were rather vague as to the future of the voluntary hospitals.

The public received the interim report with interest and some enthusiasm. The ideas followed current thinking by the medical profession and also redeemed the pledges made in Lloyd George's election manifesto. Lord Dawson addressed many branch meetings of the BMA and received almost unanimous support. Towards the end of 1920, a number of medical men began to have doubts. These chiefly concerned payment and could probably have been resolved. But, in the middle of 1920, the Minister of Health found himself confronted by a crisis which threatened to destroy the whole structure of British medicine.

In April 1920 Lord Knutsford, chairman of the London Hospital, bluntly told the Government that the voluntary hospitals would be unable to continue work unless the Exchequer provided one-third of their income. The hospitals had tried to raise funds by various methods, some bizarre, but had been defeated by rising prices. In the summer a number of hospitals found it necessary to close beds, the London Fever Hospital reported that it could no longer continue, and the National Hospital, Queen Square, discharged patients preparatory to closing. Radical reform of medicine was now out of the question; the Minister found it necessary to devote his entire energy to saving the situation. He raised £700,000 from the National Relief Fund and persuaded King Edward's Hospital Fund to make a capital grant of £250,000. This sum, although barely sufficient to meet the accumulated hospital debt, at least staved off the crisis. Dr Addison introduced his Bill, implementing the Maclean Report, against this background. The Bill scraped through the Commons, only to be defeated in the Lords. When re-introduced, all clauses relating to hospital reform had been dropped. A magnificent opportunity was lost and, as it transpired, lost for ever. Dawson's scheme would have integrated general practitioner with consultant, curative medicine with preventive.

Applied at first only to the wage-earner, the scope could gradually have been extended until it embraced all classes and evolved into a true National Health Service.

In 1924 a great although now almost forgotten Minister of Health named Neville Chamberlain took office. Chamberlain decided on radical reform of the Poor Law. He studied the question carefully and in November 1928 presented his Local Government Bill. The Bill empowered, but did not force, local authorities to acquire Poor Law infirmaries. Many, notably the London County Council, took advantage of the powers granted under the Act. The old Poor Law or Asylums Board hospitals were swiftly upgraded until the standard of sick care approached that of the large voluntary hospitals. Cooperation between the two types of hospital rapidly increased. By the mid-1930s the majority of 'honoraries' attached to voluntary hospitals also held a paid 'consultant' post at a municipal institution. The teaching hospital 'honorary' often took his firm of students to the municipal hospital where the student benefited by seeing a type of patient not often found in the teaching wards. Cooperation had become so close by the outbreak of the Second World War that many doctors and administrators thought the future of the hard-pressed voluntary hospitals lay in the hands of local government.

Meanwhile, a new plan of voluntary insurance against hospital charges had come into operation. It will be remembered that the Hospital Saturday Fund originated as a means of raising money for hospitals and that subscribers later claimed the right to free treatment. In 1922 King Edward's Hospital Fund for London produced a scheme designed to help voluntary hospitals in their difficulties. Available to anyone earning less than £6 a week, the plan offered free hospital treatment in return for a subscription of 3d. a week or 12s. a year. The scheme was administered by a body known as the Hospital Savings Association. Although fiercely opposed by the Labour Party, the Trade Unions and the Hospital Saturday Fund on the grounds that 'private' patients, i.e. subscribers to HSA, would receive preferential treatment, this became a popular method of insurance. Many large firms made a bulk payment to cover all their employees. HSA contained an element of charity in that a number of people subscribed without the intention of making use of the benefits offered. By 1939 all hospital patients, except the truly destitute, were paying some part of their maintenance costs either through a scheme or by direct payments arranged with the almoner.

The Government anticipated that the Second World War would bring immediate air raids, requiring hospital accommodation for at least 30,000 casualties in the first week. The Emergency Medical Service was organized as 'sectors'. Hospitals in danger areas became casualty clearing stations, patients being evacuated after emergency treatment to institutions in safer districts. In London, believed to be the main target of attack, a teaching hospital formed the apex of each sector, casualties being evacuated to large asylums and other hospitals in the country. The apex hospital was entirely cleared of ordinary sick and manned by a skeleton staff. Ordinary sick were treated in local government hospitals, which also acted as receiving stations in emergency. Bombing did not occur on the anticipated scale and, although the emergency service became very hard pressed at times, the full sector organization never came into operation. The scheme was a good one and, if applied to normal peacetime conditions, might have brought order into the chaos of voluntary and local government hospital services. Many doctors foresaw a complex headed by the central teaching hospital and stretching into the periphery. City hospitals, sited in areas largely composed of shops and offices, drew their patients from dormitory suburbs. The peripheral hospital, forming part of the central teaching institution, would attract patients from the local catchment area. Thus the patient would benefit from the upgrading of a hospital which lay closer to his home. Staff and students would also benefit from a much wider experience.

But the special conditions of warfare necessitated other and more radical changes in medicine. Obviously, the massive production of wounds must influence methods of treatment. Continuous irrigation of shell injuries with bland antiseptics was introduced by Alexis Carrel and Henry Dakin in 1915. Rest by immobilization of severely wounded areas dates from 1918, a technique greatly advanced by Joseph Trueta in the Spanish Civil War. The urgent need to find a safe method of combating infection instigated work on penicillin at the beginning of the Second World War. Surgery of the lung and brain was almost non-existent until experience of battle casualties in 1914—18 opened up a wide and hopeful field of endeavour. Plastic surgery owes far more to the wartime work of Harold Delf Gillies and Archibald McIndoe than to any discoveries made in time of peace. Treatment and repair of extensive burns met with little success until the Second World War. Prevention and reversal of shock was immensely improved by experience gained in the First World War. Blood transfusion, tentatively used at the first battle of Cambrai in 1917, did not become a routine procedure until familiarity with air-raid casualties in 1940 showed that resuscitation, the recovery of shocked and injured patients to a state fit for operation, could not be successful until a volume of blood almost equal to that lost had been replaced. Other and less specialized benefits deriving from warfare are the Red Cross organizations which date from Henri Dunant's publication in 1862 of the horrors witnessed at the battle of Solferino, and the improvement in nursing partly attributable to the example of Florence Nightingale in the Crimean War of 1854.

Such are a few of the medical advances which must, rather unwillingly, be attributed to war. But the most significant discovery, and that which radically altered the function of the army doctor, is the essential need of efficient sanitation and uncontaminated water supply in campaign conditions. Until the twentieth century it was commonplace for more soldiers to die from disease than from wounds. The organisms responsible for typhoid and dysentery had been discovered before the Boer War of 1899—1901 and measures for prevention, including anti-typhoid inoculation, were available. But the army lacked sanitary discipline; the surgeon was still a 'wound-doctor' rather than an officer whose orders must be obeyed. Thus, despite all advances in knowledge, 6,425 British soldiers died of wounds and 11,327 of disease in the last year of the war. The number of typhoid cases alone amounted to 42,741, just over a tenth of the total troops engaged. In the Russo-Japanese War of 1904—5 both sides imposed strict sanitary and water discipline. The Japanese lost 58,357 men by enemy action and 21,802 from disease. The Russians did not release casualty figures but claimed that only 7,960 died from sickness, about one-hundredth of the army on active service. The Russo-Japanese is the first war in which disease took a lesser toll than wounds.

The function of an army doctor had changed by 1914. He was no longer a semi-civilian who treated illness and wounds as they occurred, but an integral part of the fighting force whose instructions must be considered by the high command and whose orders must be obeyed by the troops. The change involved a new doctor—patient relationship, because in civilian life a patient retains freedom of choice and also because a large part of the population had been conscripted into the ranks and were therefore subordinate. The point is well illustrated by a story dating from the First World War. A private reported sick to the medical officer. 'Look here, my man, if we were in civilian life would you come to my surgery with a trivial complaint like this?' 'Of course not, sir. I should send for you.' This changed relationship applied not only to the armed services but also to a section of the civilian population during the Second World War. Air-raid casualties, dug out of their bombed homes, were not asked which doctor they would like to visit or whether they preferred to be treated privately in a nursing home. They were taken by ambulance to the nearest reception centre and seen by the medical officer on duty. In this respect the war effected a minor social revolution.

There were a number of doctors at the end of the Second World War who had experienced the authority necessarily invested in them by service in the armed forces. There were a number of laymen who had submitted to medical dictates rendered necessary by warfare and who had resigned their freedom of choice whether as service personnel or as civilians. The wars had effected a certain 'Teutonization' of medicine, a doctor—patient relationship more akin to that traditional in Germany than to that which obtained in peacetime Britain. Taking these points into consideration, it is possible to explain the general agreement between doctors and laymen that some kind of National Health Service must necessarily emerge as part of post-war reconstruction after both World Wars. Acceptance of regimentation by conscription and rationing, a closer integration of social classes, the need for combined effort rather than for individual exertion, may also be cited as phenomena common to both wars and tending to suggest public responsibility for the welfare of all people. The need for a Health Service was generally admitted but the form which the Service should take caused acute divergence of opinion.

10 A Health Service in being

Lloyd George had the example of Bismarck's Germany before his eyes when he introduced National Health Insurance in 1911. Those who sought to frame a National Health Service in the 1940s had little experience upon which to draw. The oldest comprehensive Health Service is that of Russia, dating from 1862. Like most Tsarist social reforms, it was good in intention but bad in practice, largely because of the vast area to be served and the shortage of well-trained personnel. 'Flying squads' of doctors and specialists visited the remoter areas at infrequent intervals but the peasant depended for his ordinary medical attention upon the *feldsher*, a semi-trained orderly rather similar to the *medicus* of the Roman legions, and who had in fact originated as a failed student of Peter the Great's medical school in Moscow. The service incorporated a measure of compulsion, since the whole village must attend the doctor on his visits. It was free to all, without insurance contributions.

The service had greatly improved by 1914 when, it is said, no Russian village lay more than thirty-two kilometres (twenty miles) from a hospital. These hospitals were small, of the cottage type and usually staffed by only one doctor who supervised all branches of medicine, often performed by semi-trained assistants. The doctor was paid by the State, through town or village council. The First World War greatly decreased the number available and scarcity continued during the first years of the Soviet regime. Soviets therefore had no option but to carry on a system which is obviously economical of skilled manpower, since one qualified member can direct and supervise a number of unqualified helpers in the field. Thus the Health Service of the USSR depended, as it depends today, upon the Health Centre or 'Polyclinic' from which all branches of medical science, curative, preventive and social, are practised and administered.

Norway, a large and mountainous country with a small scattered population, is believed to have appointed government paid employees, who were not necessarily medically qualified, in charge of public health and of patient care. This rudimentary service existed many years ago and, at the end of the nineteenth century, developed as an insurance scheme with free hospital treatment. Sweden, another sparsely populated country, also introduced a form of Health Service early in the twentieth century, when a National Board of Health appointed provincial physicians to act as a combination of general practitioner and public health officer. The Swedish service is also based upon insurance but is not entirely 'free' since the patient must pay his doctor and recover a proportion of the fee from national insurance. Germany combined health insurance with an Imperial Health Department, founded before 1880, the officers of which, known as *Kreisphysicus*, acted as district physicians and public health officers in a manner similar to those of Sweden. The continental hospital system differed from the British in that the majority, and all the larger hospitals, were 'public charities' as in France, or 'state institutions' as in Sweden, Germany and Russia.

Britain did not have the problem of small communities sparsely scattered over a difficult terrain which had dictated the development of medical services in Russia, Norway and Sweden. Nor did Britain have the long tradition of a paternalist central bureaucracy which had made a partially state-employed medical profession, with ranks and precedence similar to the civil service, acceptable in Germany. Above all, the various branches of medicine had tended to drift apart in Britain. Curative medicine lay in the hands of the general practitioner, who attended patients in his surgery or their own homes, and of the specialist, who conducted the main part of his practice in hospital ward and outpatient clinic. Preventive and social medicine was controlled almost entirely by local authorities through the Medical Officer of Health and his department. In addition, there still existed a division in the hospital service, one section depending upon voluntary subscriptions and payment by patients, the other upon compulsory rates levied by borough and county councils. In the first, the doctor was an 'honorary', giving his services freely; in the second, he was a paid servant of the local authority.

Proposals had already been made to end this separation of branches and this dual control of hospitals, but the difficulties had proved too great and they had never been implemented. On the one hand, both doctors and voluntary hospitals feared domination by local councils. On the other, the powerful and power-loving town halls saw no good reason to surrender an important part of their function. Only a solution of these problems, acceptable to all, could produce a comprehensive and efficient Health Service of the kind envisaged by Lord Dawson in his Primary and Secondary Health Centres.

It is of historical interest that the medical profession outlined the first plan, or conglomeration of plans, accepted as a basis for discussion by the BMA in 1942. The annual representative meeting passed by a small majority that a free medical service ought to be provided for the whole community, but that anyone should have the right to contract out. The meeting did not discuss reorganization of hospitals. Group practices, arranged by the doctors, and Health Centres were to be an essential of the Service. A large majority voted against whole-time salaried employment. Later in 1942 a group of younger doctors proposed a free health service for the whole population as part of a comprehensive social security scheme. Their Service was to be administered by a national corporation operating through eleven regional bodies, a plan rather similar to the war-time sectors. They proposed that both voluntary and local government hospitals remain untouched for the present, except in so far that finance and appointment of medical staff should be handled by the corporation. But, in course of time, the corporation would acquire ownership of all hospitals.

The Communist Party, the Liberals, the Labour Party, the latter in close conjunction with the Socialist Medical Association, all evolved their own schemes for a National Health Service. The Labour plan is of impor-tance, not only because the party ultimately introduced a Service, but because their solution of hospital chaos injected one of the major contro-versies into the discussion. Briefly, Labour envisaged that 'before long voluntary hospitals will come under the control of the Local Authorities'. This was exactly what the majority of the medical profession most feared.

Meanwhile, Sir William Beveridge and a committee of civil servants had been working on the subject. Beveridge published his famous report in December 1942. He assumed that there would be a comprehensive National Health Service, including hospital treatment, freely available for the whole population and financed by insurance contributions. A new form of social insurance would cover all income groups and therefore free medical treatment would be available for everyone. Beveridge disarmed criticism by drawing a parallel with education. Just as education was already free to all yet many parents opted to pay fees, so private treatment of the sick could still exist under his plan. Payment of contributions would be compulsory but acceptance of benefit would not. In February 1943 the Council of the BMA agreed to the scheme on two conditions. The character, terms and conditions of service must be negotiated with the medical profession and fee-paying patients must not be debarred from hospital treatment. In the same month Parliament accepted the report, emphasizing that benefit would not be forced upon those who preferred to make private arrangements. Thus, at the end of February 1943, both Government and medical profession had committed themselves to the principle of a National Health Service.

The Minister of Health, Mr Ernest Brown, initiated a series of secret discussions with representatives of voluntary hospitals, local authorities and the medical profession in June 1943. The discussions were exploratory and not intended to be decisive. The Minister circulated a draft paper out-lining a proposal to employ general practitioners as salaried officers in a comprehensive Service. This secret paper, nothing more than a tentative proposal for discussion, leaked into the public press, probably through the indiscretion of a medical representative. The BMA hastily called a meeting of their Metropolitan Counties branch, attended by about 1,000 doctors. Dr Charles Hill, deputy secretary of the BMA, made an inflammatory speech accusing the Government of the intention to control the medical profession and purposely destroy traditional practice by forcing the family doctor to work entirely from Health Centres.

The rights and wrongs of this disastrous incident will probably be never correctly assessed. There is no good reason to suppose that Charles Hill was accurate in his contention although he may perhaps have had inside information that this was government policy at the time. Nor is there any reason to suppose that the offensive document was anything more than an item for debate. But the harm had been done. Government intentions became suspect and the term 'Health Centre' synonymous with full-time service. It was in this atmosphere of suspicion that Mr Henry Willink, who succeeded Ernest Brown at the Ministry of Health, introduced his White Paper in February 1944. He tried to soothe fears by declaring his intention 'to use and absorb the experience of past and present, building it into a wider service'. The general practitioner would be retained, but some would be encouraged to form group practices and to work from Health Centres. Those who opted for the Health Centre might or might not be full-time salaried officers. Willink proposed that voluntary hospitals remain untouched. In order to provide a free service, local authorities must compensate for loss of patients' fees by payments to the hospitals. All hospitals, voluntary or municipal, would receive exchequer grants paid through the local authority. Honorary staff would be salaried as either full- or part-time employees. The administrative apparatus, headed by the Minister, depended upon coordination between advisory committees (Health Service Councils) consisting largely of nominated or elected doctors and the existing local government.

Willink clearly stated during the debate on the White Paper that the Government had no intention of introducing a full-time salaried service. His statement was promptly challenged. General practitioners, speaking through the BMA, now regarded any mention of Health Centres as being evidence of future evolution into full-time salaried employment. The voluntary hospital staffs feared control by local authorities. In the summer of 1944 the British Hospitals Association came out strongly against the relevant section of the Paper, claiming that hospitals would rapidly become subservient to local councils if the latter held the purse strings. The Association demanded direct exchequer grants. The jealous local authorities, speaking through the powerful London County Council, declined to accept nominated or appointed professional members on any committee charged with administration of a health scheme. Willink vainly tried to break the impasse with various concessions but found himself in an impossible position by July 1945. A month later the electorate declined to return their wartime hero Mr Winston Churchill to power. Mr Clement Attlee's Labour Party came back to Westminster with an overwhelming majority. Mr Attlee entrusted the Ministry of Health to Mr Aneurin Bevan.

The name of Aneurin Bevan must be accorded a very high place in any social history of medicine. But we must not forget his predecessors, Edwin Chadwick, John Simon, David Lloyd George, Lord Dawson of Penn, Lord Addison among others. We should also spare a thought for the pioneers, men like the almost forgotten Thomas Beddoes, Robert Philip and Pendrill Varrier-Jones, who first conceived curative, preventive and social medicine to be one and the same. Nor is Bevan the 'Architect of the

National Health Service', a title sometimes given to him. His Act was the culmination of twenty-eight years labour, during which many plans had been drawn and the foundations laid. To continue the architectural metaphor, Bevan is more properly described as the Builder who managed to get his tender accepted.

Bevan succeeded where others had failed. His success derived in part from his traits of character, bad as well as good. A Welshman, born of poor parents, he started his career as a miner and saw the despair caused by unemployment in the Welsh valleys. He climbed to a position of influence in the Labour Party by sheer hard work and force of character. His electorate trusted him for his integrity and for the courage with which he declared his strongly socialist opinions. Something of a statesman, he suffered from the defect of being an outstandingly able politician. Astute in debate and a master of repartee, he was too prone to vent intemperate remarks and sometimes showed little skill in diplomacy or conciliation. He served as Minister in a Government which, like its predecessor, had committed itself to the introduction of a National Health Service. The form which the Service would take did not differ greatly from that outlined in Willink's White Paper. Labour, supported by the Socialist Medical Association, favoured a full-time salaried Service to cover 100 per cent of the population. A large section of the Party, headed by Herbert Morrison, advocated integration with local authorities, both doctors and hospitals to be directed and administered from county halls. But the proposed subservience of working doctors did not accord with one of the primary objects in the Labour election manifesto, greater participation of the worker in the management of his trade. Bevan clarified his own view at his first meeting with the medical profession 'I want for the miners, the engineers, the railwaymen, a far greater share in the management of their work and the policies that govern it, and I say no less for the doctors.'

Bevan exerted all his considerable charm at this first meeting and did much to reassure those who had been terrified by the appointment of a left-wing Minister of Health. The doctors prepared for a long series of negotiations. Bevan replied that he was not prepared to waste time by retravelling all the ground covered in the past year. He reinforced this decision with a most interesting constitutional doctrine which had never been raised before. Negotiations must be meaningless unless outside bodies were informed of proposals before they had been submitted to the House of Commons. Further, negotiating implied the granting of concessions, and any concession might tie the Minister's hands when dealing with amendments proposed by the House. His attitude was undoubtedly correct but resulted in renewed suspicion of his good intentions.

In November 1945, within two months of taking office, the press reported that Bevan had drafted an outline plan and had received Cabinet sanction. A spate of rumours followed which included the account—probably true—of wide divergence of opinion within the Labour Party hierarchy. Bevan published his White Paper in March 1946. Surprisingly, he had thrown overboard many doctrinaire socialist ideas on the future of hospitals. Instead of turning over all hospitals to the local authorities, he proposed to appropriate both voluntary and municipal hospitals and to administer them by regional boards consisting of members chosen and appointed by the Minister. The boards, in turn, were to appoint management committees, after consultation with local authorities, medical and dental staffs, for each large hospital or group of smaller hospitals. Existing endowments would be handed over to a central fund controlled by the Ministry and apportioned among regional boards. Thus the local authority would no longer participate in provision or administration of hospitals unless elected as individual members of committees.

Bevan's proposals with regard to teaching hospitals were even more surprising. These received special treatment. They did not form part of the regional structure, although the location and number of teaching hospitals determined the fixing of regional boundaries. They were to be administered by separate boards of governors for each hospital or associated group. A board of governors included members nominated by the University, the regional board, and the senior medical staff of the hospital. Teaching hospitals were allowed to retain and to administer their endowment funds. Bevan accepted the principle of part-time service and private practice. Consultants (the new term for the old honorary staff) could elect to be either full- or part-time employees, and the latter would receive a salary based on the number of hours worked for the Service. The part-time consultant would be permitted to engage in private practice outside these hours. Further, he would be allowed fee-paying patients in Health Service hospitals. Many hospitals now possessed private wings, and these would not be touched. Bevan justified this concession in words which are relevant today 'unless we permit some fee-paying patients in the public hospitals, there will be a rash of nursing homes all over the country'.

The general practitioner and dentist did not fare quite so well. They came under the control of new bodies known as executive councils, similar to the 1911 insurance committees. The councils were to be composed of equal numbers of professional members and laymen. Bevan hoped that general practitioners would agree to operate from Health Centres, to be provided by local authorities. They would retain their practices and receive a salary as well as capitation fees. But directly the Act came into operation, there would be a restriction upon doctors proposing to start a new practice in 'popular' areas. Practices would no longer be saleable. The Exchequer made £66 million available to compensate doctors for the capital already invested, but no payment from the fund would be made until death or retirement.

The bulk of preventive and social medicine remained in the hands of local authorities who would be responsible for provision and maintenance of maternity services, child welfare, health visiting, home nursing, home helps and ambulances. The proposed Bill promised a great extension of these services.

Bevan's White Paper, embodied as a Bill, passed through Parliament with only minor amendments. During the debates, Bevan was enticed into one of his more unfortunate pieces of repartee, and it has never been ascertained whether he was speaking seriously or indulging his impish sense of humour. A member of the opposition accused him of the intention to introduce a full-time salaried service, if not now at least in the future. Bevan replied 'I do not believe the medical profession is ripe for it. There is all the difference in the world between plucking fruit when it is ripe and plucking it when it is green.' It is hardly necessary to add that this remarkable utterance aroused the most acute suspicion among the medical profession. The Third Reading of the Bill passed by a large majority and it was approved by the House of Lords. Royal Assent followed on 6 November 1946 when the Bill became law. Considerable spade work would be necessary before implementation and the appointed day was fixed for 5 July 1948.

Unlike his predecessors, Bevan had clearly seen that he could not satisfy everyone. He had deliberately jettisoned a fair amount of socialist dogma. A far more astute politician than any doctor, he set out to gain the support of the most influential part of the profession. Since the Councils of Royal Colleges are largely drawn from teaching hospitals, he gave the teaching hospitals preference and worked closely with leading members of the Colleges rather than with the British Medical Association. His tactics can be exemplified in what must be called the Legend of the Merit Awards—legend because only two men knew the truth of what happened. Bevan insisted that all consultants, whatever their speciality, should be paid at the same basic rate. This thoroughly annoyed the proud physician and surgeon, who were affronted that their services should be valued at the same price as the radiologist who took 'their' X-rays and the anaesthetist who gave 'their' anaesthetics. The disagreement became formidable. The Spens Committee, set up in 1947 to consider the remuneration of medical staff, suggested a system of merit or distinction awards for consultants who did particularly brilliant work in their specialities. Legend has it that Bevan dined with Lord Moran, President of the Royal College of Physicians, at Prunier's Restaurant in St James's Street. During the course of dinner he handed over control of a large secret fund to Lord Moran to share out in the form of distinction awards *in any way that Lord Moran and two colleagues decided best.* Whether the legend be true or not, there is no doubt that for a number of years Lord Moran and his two colleagues did distribute merit awards in circumstances of great secrecy—and the 'ancillary specialities' came off very badly.

Bevan drove a wedge between the hospital consultant and the general practitioner. He deliberately made use of the long-lived split in the medical profession. Lord Dawson, a statesman and a physician, had sought to heal the breach by drawing the general practitioner into closer contact with the hospital. Bevan may be said to have made the divorce absolute. Even the small cottage hospitals were ultimately to be taken out of the family doctor's hands. For the present he remained a member of the staff in a kind of second-rate consultant grade known as a Senior Hospital Medical Officer, but he would be gradually phased out when a sufficient number of consultants had been trained to take his place. The hospital doctor, particularly the teaching hospital consultant, did very well out of Bevan's Act. His private practice remained unaffected. He was now paid for the work which he had previously done for nothing. He received valuable emoluments, travelling expenses, six weeks paid holiday a year, generous periods of 'study leave'. Bevan cynically admitted that he had resorted to bribery. 'I have stuffed their mouths with gold' he told a friend.

The general practitioner found little attractive in the Act. He disliked the proposal that local authorities should provide Health Centres as the foci of practice. Many foresaw a day when they would be salaried full-time officers controlled by county hall. They feared domination by the local authority more than anything else, for councils had a bad record in their treatment of medical staff. They feared direction, seeing the clause which required a doctor to obtain permission before starting a new practice in certain areas as the hidden intention to order him to work in the less attractive districts. They did not trust the semi-confiscation of their practices with a promise of compensation at some remote date. They suspected the basic salary, an emolument of £300 a year primarily designed to help the young man until he had become established, as being the first step towards abolition of capitation fees and so of the patient's right to choose his own doctor.

The public on the whole welcomed the new Act. They found it hard to understand why the doctors objected to terms which seemed generous. The bitter and rather unseemly wrangle which now developed between doctors and government was translated by public opinion into a squalid attempt to extract more money. In fact this was quite incorrect. The Spens Committee, surveying the period 1936—8, came to the conclusion that the majority of doctors had been grossly underpaid. Over 40 per cent in the age group 40—55, their peak earning years, received an income of less than £1,000 per annum. By accepting the Health Service terms, the 'average' general practitioner would enjoy a much higher income than he could have expected before. It is virtually impossible to define their exact grounds of objection. The intentions of the Minister were suspect. It was future policy rather than the present structure of the Service which aroused alarm.

The BMA conducted a poll on the question 'Shall we or shall we not enter into any discussion on the framework to be created within the limitation of this Act?' About 90 per cent of doctors replied. Sixty-four per cent of general practitioners answered in the negative but only 55 per cent of hospital specialists voted 'No'. A representative meeting endorsed this reply by 252 votes to 17. The Council of the BMA more or less declared open war upon the Government, choosing the weapons of propaganda and refusal to cooperate. The Council declared that the whole medical profession would decline to serve unless the Act was modified.

The ensuing struggle lasted for the first five months of 1948. Aneurin Bevan at first appeared aloof and calm, contenting himself with the hope that before reaching a final decision 'wiser counsels will have prevailed'. As tempers mounted, he bitterly resented the many attacks made on his integrity, and his gift for pungent repartee led him into a number of intemperate remarks which only served to inflame his opponents. The profession, and the BMA in particular, behaved badly. They found difficulty in propounding a rational argument for, as has already been mentioned, antagonism depended more upon intuition than upon reason. In such circumstances, vituperation is more likely than calm discussion. The writer well remembers that it required moral courage and even some physical bravery to state a case for the Service at meetings determined to insist upon a solid front of opposition. Support for the BMA poured in from general practitioners all over the country. The BMA, anxious to represent a united profession, wooed the hospital medical staffs. Hospital 'honoraries' were not quite happy that the promises made to them would be kept. (Incidentally, their fears were justified. Thirty years later a Minister of Health declared her intention to 'phase out' private beds.) At specially convened meetings of their medical committees, they declared their unanimous support for the BMA. The support was not quite so unanimous as the resolutions suggested. At one teaching hospital some half-dozen members of the staff boldly protested. The chairman then put the motion 'The Medical Board of X Hospital unanimously agree that they will not accept service under the terms of the present Act.' The half-dozen recalcitrants duly voted against the proposal but, being carried by a majority, it went forward as a 'unanimous' decision. There is reason to believe that many hospital committees adopted this rather unusual procedure. Always before the BMA was the fiasco of 1911. In the words of their Chairman, Dr H. Guy Dain, 'we have better organization now, and we will jolly well see it does not happen this time'. A poll conducted by the BMA in February 1948, answered by 84 per cent of doctors, showed that 90 per cent of these disapproved of the Act and that 88 per cent would not accept service. Less than 4,000, a number quite insufficient to make the Health Service viable, were prepared to accept the terms.

On 7 April Bevan made one of the cleverest speeches ever to be delivered in the House of Commons. He adopted a very conciliatory attitude. He gave way on one or two minor points while remaining adamant upon essentials. His most surprising 'peace proposal' was the offer to sponsor a statutory provision designed to *prohibit* a full-time salaried service. His slight and partial surrenders carried much less weight than the whole matter and manner of his speech. He was so friendly, so sympathetic towards the problems of the doctors, as to leave the impression that he appreciated their justifiable suspicion and desired nothing more than to reassure them. The British Medical Association's faith in the justice of their cause was somewhat shaken but they considered that professional freedom was still not adequately protected. Bevan's concessions were such that the Association decided on another referendum later in April. Only 77 per cent of doctors replied, perhaps an indication that they were tired of polls rather than that they had been reassured by Bevan. Analysis showed resistance to be crumbling. Although a large majority still disapproved of the Act, fewer than 10,000 doctors opposed service. The BMA required at least 13,000 to make resistance effective.

At this point Dr Alfred Cox, who had been medical secretary of the BMA in 1911, decided it was time to give his advice. He reminded the BMA of their humiliating defeat over Lloyd George's Insurance Act. He pointed out that this inglorious surrender had been caused by the action of a few die-hards who decided to hold out while thousands of doctors were 'flocking to the panel'. Cox strongly advised the Council of the BMA to approve the Act before resistance dwindled to such an extent as to leave them virtually isolated. Bevan seized the opportunity to write a conciliatory letter. He did little more than reiterate his promises of 7 April which he proposed to embody in an amending Bill. The Council called a special Representative Meeting on 28 May.

This meeting, perhaps the most momentous in the history of the BMA, produced an acrimonious but on the whole well-reasoned debate. Representatives made charges that the Council had no authority to hold the April referendum, that it was premature, and had 'split the profession far more effectively than Mr Bevan could have dreamed of doing'. Thirty-eight per cent of representatives demanded the Council's resignation. The Chairman, Dr Dain, made a skilful defence in which he claimed that the majority of desired concessions had been won. On the question of good intention, he pointed out that Ministers of Health had kept faith with the profession for a quarter of a century. He then dealt with the doctors' attitude. Some, he said, would oppose a National Health Service of any form or kind. These could not be placated. Many more genuinely desired a comprehensive Health Service. They might object to certain parts of the Act but they wanted the Service as a whole. This section of Dain's speech is of particular interest because, although perhaps not remarked at the time, he was reminding his colleagues that the original demand for a Health Service and the first plans had come from the doctors themselves.

In spite of a fighting and hotly angry speech from Lord Horder, a convinced opponent of any kind of State medicine, the majority of representatives faced up to reality and supported the Council's resolution to accept the Act. Bevan's letter had done the trick. The Council was able to greet his promise of an amending Bill as a major victory. It may have been a notable victory or it may not. The Council was probably more impressed by the fact that a quarter of all doctors in Britain had already accepted the terms offered and many more had announced their intention of doing so. But at least the British Medical Association could bow itself out with dignity. The 'humiliating retreat' of 1912 had been avoided.

Aneurin Bevan won his battle and the National Health Service came into operation on the day appointed, 5 July 1948. That is certain. It is not so certain that the changes effected can be properly described as a National Health Service. Care of the sick formed only part of a much larger scheme, a system of social security protecting the citizen from his cradle (maternity benefit) to his grave (contribution towards funeral expenses). We are here concerned only with those parts which affected the practice of medicine. There was no attempt to follow Dawson's plan for Primary and Secondary Health Centres, a means of absorbing general practitioner and consultant into a coherent organization. Even the proposed 'Health Centres' were tacitly dropped. A very few came into being on an experimental basis, but family doctors much preferred to work from their own surgeries. The Act did nothing to integrate preventive with curative medicine, while social medicine remained the prerogative of the town hall. In a true 'Health Service' the consultant does not dwell apart in a hospital, to be called on an occasional domiciliary visit when the practitioner is troubled and the patient unfit to be moved. He is close at hand to advise. Equally, the general practitioner does not dismiss everything requiring hospital care to the consultant. He has his own beds and operating theatre where he can undertake the care of such patients as he is competent to treat. Above all, the machinery of preventive medicine is closely linked to that of curative. All ranks of the profession, without exception, are left in no doubt that it is their primary duty to prevent disease rather than to attempt a belated cure. None of these desiderata exist in the National Health Service as at present constituted. The hospitals are 'nationalized' but, for the rest, our Health Service is little more than a comprehensive scheme of national insurance.

The 1946 Act brought undoubted benefits to the majority of patients. Not the worker only but his whole family could now attend doctor and dentist free of charge. The change-over proceeded smoothly despite gloomy prophecies of chaos. Within a few weeks, Bevan found it necessary to make an appeal for moderation in the use of his Service. There had always been hospital waiting lists, over-crowded doctors' surgeries, a shortage of personnel. These deficiencies were intensified by increased willingness of the public to visit the doctor and dentist, perhaps stimulated by a natural desire to receive full value for the weekly insurance contribution. This had one curious result. The state of the nation's teeth was collectively rotten. School clinics had effected some improvement but only the more wealthy class wasted money on a visit to the dentist unless in acute pain. In 1948 dentistry temporarily became the most highly-paid profession in Britain. Dentists, paid on the basis of each procedure carried out, had more work than they could conveniently do.

No question of possible payments now arose when a patient entered hospital. The almoner could concentrate on the more pleasant and useful part of her work, helping patients in difficulty, rather than badgering them for contributions towards maintenance. The old-time Housekeeping Sister gave place to a well-qualified Catering Officer who, freed from the urgent need for strict economy, provided a much better standard of cooking and food. Hospitals found it possible to relax many irksome rules and regulations, which had often been necessarily introduced because of staff shortage. Amenity funds, a grant of money separate from the ordinary hospital budget, were used to brighten up and refurnish dull waiting rooms, corridors and wards. The hospital became better equipped with modern apparatus, to the improvement of diagnosis and treatment. Above all, the patient no longer had the sense of being an object of charity in a voluntary hospital or a pauper in a municipal infirmary. He had paid for his stay in the ward by insurance contributions and he was part-owner of the nationalized hospital. Where before a complaint might be met with an admonition to be thankful, he could now express his views with some certainty that they would receive attention. And he often did so. Many of the reforms and improvements in hospital life have resulted from a patient's criticism.

The doctors found that their lives went on very much as before. One serious objection to a comprehensive Health Service had been that a patient might not only demand his right to treatment but also his right to dictate the form of treatment given. A number of doctors, particularly consultants, expected to be faced with this difficulty after the appointed day. There is no evidence that patients proved any more 'difficult' than before. By the end of the first year, it became apparent that the Service was working satisfactorily but it also became apparent that many more doctors and nurses were needed and that there was a grave shortage of hospital beds. These problems could not be solved at once. Britain was going through a period of financial difficulty and had little cash to spare. But, given time and a sounder economy, increase of staff and new hospital building would be possible. Of course other troubles developed. General practitioners, now dependent on fixed capitation fees for the major part of their incomes, found purchasing value eroded by inflation and demanded an increase. Hospital consultants, particularly when full-time and paid fixed salaries, found their incomes falling in terms of real money. Such troubles, although productive of angry storms and threats of industrial action, were minor matters which could be and were adjusted by arbitration.

The Health Service worked. But the Government, the public, and many doctors overlooked one essential point. The Service only worked because of inherited good will and almost any system, however bad, can be made to function if all are willing. We must remember that every doctor is trained in a medical school and that, until 1948, all medical schools were attached to voluntary hospitals. The student was 'reared in the spirit of the voluntary hospital'. Voluntary hospitals ran on a shoestring. The hospital could only exist if everyone was prepared to help. Everything non-essential to the patient's welfare had to be cut to a minimum. A hospital of 500 beds employing an equal number of staff in their various duties might be administered by a secretary, an assistant secretary, and one typist. Other departments such as the steward's, the salaries office, the engineer's, were staffed on the same kind of scale. The senior 'honoraries' not only gave their services free of charge, but made large contributions from their own pockets in times of need. House surgeons rarely had any fixed off-time or holidays and were paid an honorarium of £50 a year. Nurses, grossly underpaid, cheerfully worked long hours and submitted themselves to strict discipline. Students willingly performed a variety of odd jobs that could not strictly be called educational, such as the routine changing of dressings and collection of blood samples. The welfare of the patient took precedence over everything else and, however great the burden on its staff, the hospital must carry out its work.

This 'voluntary hospital spirit' was not a discipline to be quickly forgotten. It did not suddenly die on 5 July 1948 but persisted for many years. Just as the spirit had carried the voluntary hospitals, so it carried the National Health Service. One cannot identify the point at which good will started to run out, for the process of erosion was gradual. The doctor found himself increasingly frustrated. Ambitious and hard working general practitioners, now debarred from the cottage hospital, found little incentive to do more than routine work. They received the same capitation fee as less conscientious doctors who barely troubled to examine their patients and sent everything that promised to be troublesome to the nearest hospital. The hospital consultant in turn became swamped with a type of illness that could have been dealt with by the general practitioner. A specialist in diseases of the liver spent long hours in the outpatient department examining patients who suffered from chronic bronchitis and similar ailments. A surgeon, skilled in the specialized science of vascular surgery, repaired hernias and removed ingrowing toenails. It was all useful work and all very necessary, but could have been done more economically by less skilled staff in Primary Health Centres had such existed. Specialized medicine and surgery continued to become more complex and more time-consuming. An E.N.T. specialist must fit an ear operation, requiring four hours' work, into a routine list of tonsillectomies and other comparatively minor procedures. The physician must somehow manage to undertake a prolonged investigation during his daily round in ward and outpatient department. The 'notional session' became meaningless; the consultant simply worked until the work was finished.

Intrusion of politics exacerbated discontent. A Green Paper and Consultative Document of 1972 appears to have had for its purpose a closer integration of preventive with curative medicine. As implemented in April 1974 the only overt effect was to make administrative machinery more cumbersome and to separate lay administration more widely from the working doctor. A hospital consultant had now to penetrate several strata of committees before arriving at the source of management. The nature of these new committees intensified the political aspect. The old friendly teacher—trainee association showed signs of strain and began to be replaced by an unhappy boss—worker relationship. Registrars, the intermediate grade through which an intending consultant must pass, no longer regarded the chief's absence as a chance to gain valuable experience. Many saw no good reason why they should do a consultant's work at a registrar's pay when the former was on holiday or attending a conference. House surgeons no longer looked upon their office as privileged training but demanded regular off-duty periods, rebelled against their over-long hours, and expected to be paid overtime. Nursing ceased to be a semi-charitable vocation and became a trade with all its modern concomitants, demonstration marches, militants, threats of strikes. Students forgot that bedside contact with patients is an essential part of their education and refused to act as laboratory assistants or nursing orderlies. Then the part-time consultants considered that the promises made to them, the terms under which they had accepted employment, were in danger of being broken and resorted to a form of industrial action. The leaders of a great and honourable profession, whose motto has always been 'the patient must come first' were forced by circumstances outside their control to act in a manner unthinkable before 1948.

What had gone wrong? Some would blame the senior doctors, holding that they are too conservative, unwilling to move with the times. Yet it is the younger generation, who never knew medicine before the Health Service, which is most actively expressing disillusionment by seeking a career in other lands. Some point to increasing interference by party politicians. But, surveying the scene in the troubled months of 1975, the causes of discontent, although perhaps unexpressed, seem to be more deeply seated than is suggested by surface disagreement. It is reasonable to suppose that there must have been faults in the original structure of the Health Service, that good will served to paper over the cracks, and that the cracks became apparent when good will had been lost. Perhaps we are passing through a transition phase from one form of medicine to another; such periods of transition are historically accompanied by convulsions. Or perhaps nationalized medicine owes too much to a way of thought dictated by the exigencies of warfare and, in its present form, is not suited to peacetime conditions. Curative medicine, although based upon science, is after all still primarily an individual art, and creative artists do not take kindly to bureaucratic control even in totalitarian states.

The International Health Service provides a rather more happy story of cooperation. Medicine has always been international or supranational in character. The application of medical science to the patient varies from country to country but the science itself is shared by all. We have already seen that this is so. Roman doctors were of Greek extraction; the School of Salerno drew students from all Western Europe and Asia Minor; Englishmen studied at Padua, Montpellier and Leyden; the great centres such as Paris and Edinburgh attracted doctors of many nationalities other than their own. This international character of medical science is well exemplified by the work done on mosquito-borne diseases during the nineteenth century. Worldwide research led to discoveries by the British workers Patrick Manson and Ronald Ross, by the French army surgeon Alphonse Laveran, by the Italians Camillo Golgi and Giovanni Grassi, by a number of Americans including Carlos Finlay and William Crawford Gorgas. The findings of all these men, working in a number of countries, added together to unravel the nature of malaria and yellow fever. The solution permitted a great international advance. Gorgas, having defeated yellow fever in the West Indies, transferred his activities to the Panama Isthmus in Central America. He transformed an area which had been a white man's grave into one having a lower annual mortality than New York or London. Completion of the Panama Canal in 1914 was rendered possible by the defeat of mosquito-borne diseases, an advance which originated from the observation by Patrick Manson of Hong Kong of filarial embryos in the body of a *Culex* mosquito in 1877.

Opening of the Panama Canal shortened the journey between the Atlantic and Pacific Oceans. Travel became easier and more rapid throughout the nineteenth century. In 1813 Napoleon granted the English scientist Humphry Davy safe conduct across Europe because he wished to study the extinct volcanoes of Auvergne and compare the geological formation with active Vesuvius, a proof that science knows no frontiers and can sometimes transcend warfare. Davy left Plymouth on 15 October and reached Paris a week later. The doctor who desired to visit Berlin or Vienna at the beginning of the nineteenth century must expect to spend weeks on the road. Travel was costly. Only a wealthy doctor of the 1830s could afford the time and money to visit a European centre. This state of affairs changed within the span of a lifetime. Steam power made travel much more rapid and cheaper in the 1870s. The doctor who desired to visit Berlin could now be back in his London consulting room within a week. An efficient postal system delivered his letters rapidly and at little cost. Improved printing methods and fast transport not only increased the number of medical journals but made them readily available in every country. Publications such as the *Lancet* carried weekly reports from correspondents in Paris, Vienna and St Petersburg. Just as the great trade exhibitions drew people from all over the world, so the doctor attended international conferences and exchanged ideas with his foreign colleagues. This increased mobility and easy exchange of information accounts for the very rapid and worldwide advance in medicine during the last quarter of the nineteenth century. Let us recapitulate the story of X-rays as an example. Röntgen communicated his discovery to the Würzburg Physico-Medical Society in a paper published in their *Proceedings* on 28 December 1895. A translation by Arthur Stanton appeared in the British journal *Nature* on 23 January 1896. Two days later, on 25 January, the *Lancet* carried photographs of a human hand and of a frog made by A. Campbell Swinton in his laboratory at 66 Victoria Street, London. On 22 February the *Lancet* published a report from Liverpool that an air-gun pellet had been localized by means of X-rays and successfully removed. Less than two months elapsed between the first report of X-rays in a journal published in South-East Germany and their first known diagnostic use in Britain.

Increased mobility did not always produce beneficial results. The first contact of one community with another may bring disaster. Plague, syphilis, cholera, and probably virulent smallpox have all reached Western Europe from exotic sources. Such has been the case since the first ships of the Mediterranean civilization made contact with Africa and the East. An epidemic on a small slowly-moving sailing vessel tended to die out during the voyage (although yellow fever was widely disseminated by mosquitoes breeding in the ship's supply of drinking water) but the rapid steamer increased the risk of carrying infection from one land to another. In 1875 a cruiser, HMS *Dido*, visited the Fiji group of islands. There was a small epidemic of measles among the crew. Nearly a quarter of the unprotected Fijiian population died within three months. The epidemic spread by sea to all the South Pacific Islands with equally devastating results. Similar disasters attended the introduction of tuberculosis and syphilis to peoples who had not experienced them before. Flying has made the danger more acute. A passenger in the incubation stage of an exotic infection can land in an unprotected country before any signs or symptoms are apparent.

International spread of illness and international exchange of information suggested international control of disease. The work at first centred on the codification of quarantine regulations, which varied greatly from country to country. This was undertaken by a conference at Paris in 1851. As knowledge of epidemiology increased, it became possible to attack problems with greater certainty. International conferences dealt with the spread of cholera in 1892—4 and with the danger of plague dissemination by Mecca pilgrims in 1897. The first organization for World Health, Office International d'Hygiène Publique, was established at Paris in 1907. The League of Nations carried on and enlarged the work by means of a Health Organization set up in 1923. This was an epidemic intelligence service at the start, operating from Geneva with branches at the Paris Office, Washington DC, Alexandria, Singapore and Sydney. The scope of activities widened to include standardization of drugs and sera. Committees studied malaria, leprosy and cancer. Rural hygiene, housing and nutrition also came under survey. One of the more important of the League's contributions to world health was the not altogether unsuccessful attempt to control traffic in drugs, particularly opium and cocaine.

The United Nations Relief and Rehabilitation Administration (UNRRA), created in 1943, acted as an international health organization for just over two years. In 1946 an International Health Conference, held in New York and attended by representatives of sixty nations, took over the functions of UNRRA and formed the permanent World Health Organization (WHO) on 7 April 1948. WHO absorbed the Paris Office and the Health Organization of the League. The centre remains at Geneva, with offices in New York to maintain contact with the parent United Nations. Regional offices deal with special questions in Africa, the Eastern Mediterranean and other areas. A multitude of problems have been attacked including malaria and venereal disease. There has been a very successful campaign against tuberculosis while smallpox has been almost defeated by a vast programme of vaccination. In 1975 Bangladesh was officially declared free from smallpox, leaving only Ethiopia as a source of infection.* Embracing as it does all medical functions, preventive, curative and social, WHO may be regarded as a Supra-National Health Service,

---

* Ethiopia was declared free of smallpox in September 1976.

having for its object 'the attainment by all peoples of the highest possible level of health', regarded as the right of everyone, irrespective of race, religion or political creed.

The ideal of 'the highest possible level of health' has not yet been attained even by the most privileged nations. Much disease is still preventible. There is, for instance, an undoubted statistical relationship between heavy cigarette smoking and cancer of the lung. Many doctors would argue that smoking, overeating and overdrinking, worry and lack of exercise contribute to the high incidence of coronary infarction. We are surrounded by potential dangers. Lassa fever, the Marburg virus and the Machupo virus are examples of localized infections which could be the cause of lethal pandemics if carried to communities which have not previously experienced them. We live by the mercy of both Nature and our fellow men. Famine and war can produce conditions in which a comparatively trivial disease will assume the character of a virulent pestilence. The obvious example is the influenza pandemic of 1918—19, which became so widely diffused that only St Helena, New Guinea and a few Pacific islands entirely escaped infection. The death toll was appalling, more than 150,000 in Britain and not less than 15 million of the world population. Yet this was 'only influenza' of a type which has probably been experienced both before and after 1918. Hunger, bad living conditions and war-weariness lowered resistance on a massive scale and so produced a worldwide mortality not experienced since the time of the Black Death.

We are endangered by medical advance itself. Iatrogenic disease is that produced by the physician. Here the obvious and terrible example is thalidomide, hailed as 'a major breakthrough', a non-addictive hypnotic so safe that it could be given to young children. Introduced in 1956, it was not until 1961 that the disastrous effects of this 'harmless' drug became apparent. For several years doctors in Germany, Australia and Britain had been puzzled by a remarkable increase in the number of cases of phocomelia, a rare but crippling deformity producing normal or rudimentary hands and feet springing directly from the trunk. Investigation revealed that these unfortunate children had been born to mothers who had taken thalidomide during early pregnancy.

This is not an isolated incident; we have already mentioned the Lübeck disaster with BCG on p. 128. But there can be no shadow of doubt that, despite occasional disasters, despite the potential dangers which still face us, the sum of medical advances has been wholly beneficial. Not only medicine in its narrow sense, for it was increase of medical knowledge which prompted the work of sanitary reformers, local authorities and Ministers of Health. The efforts of all these have combined to give us a cleaner and more healthy life. This better life has altered the pattern of death. In so doing, it has brought us face to face with the new problem of old age.

Until little over a century ago the great killers were still the bacterial or zymotic infections: tuberculosis, cholera, typhus, enteric fevers, and the 'childish' diseases. These struck at all age groups and to them must be added an infantile mortality which destroyed one-sixth of all children in the first year of life. A disease pattern of this kind produced a short average life-span; the average age of death stood at forty-five years in 1850. These infections are not only less common today, because of improved methods of prevention, but will respond to treatment and so are rarely fatal. Average life expectation has therefore risen and stands today at seventy-two years. The killing diseases of the present time are the degenerative processes of cardiac and respiratory systems, arteriosclerosis, coronary infarcts and the cancers. All these disorders existed a century ago but were regarded as natural terminations because over-average span of life started in the forty-sixth year. It is only recently that death from cancer or a coronary infarct in the fifth decade has been considered an avoidable tragedy. This is simply because a man of forty-five today is still in early middle-age; he can expect a further twenty-seven years of life. In 1850 a man of forty-five was starting to enter his old age.

In 1850 the 'useless mouths' which had to be filled by the efforts of others were virtually confined to the lower age group, children who had not yet started work. The task of supporting the elderly was almost negligible. Today the average retiring age from productive work is sixty-five and rather more than one-tenth of the population of the United Kingdom is aged sixty-five or over. The age of starting work has risen since 1850; now about one-fifth of the population is below that age. The ratio of productive to non-productive is therefore 7 : 3. But this is not the whole story. Obviously, the proportion of elderly people will continue to rise and there is no reason to suppose that we have yet reached the maximum average life expectancy. It has been forecast that by 1985 the proportion of productive to non-productive citizens in USA will be as low as 13 : 14.3.

It is therefore obvious that longevity raises problems and that these problems may become more acute within the foreseeable future. But the problem is not simply that of an ever-increasing number of old people who are incapable of earning a living and who must be supported by the efforts of others. There are many who suffer from the disabilities of old age and who cannot fend for themselves. Others have out-lived their relations and their friends and cannot integrate with a younger generation; they are lonely and suffer neglect. Others are bored, without occupation for mind or body. They have lived into old age because medical advance and the social reforms prompted by medical advance have allowed them to do so, but medicine cannot make them happy. The doctor must play his part, but he can do little or nothing to bestow a healthy, contented and rewarding life upon the elderly without the aid of others, be they voluntary helpers, social workers, local authorities or Ministers of the Crown. Here, in this one example of the aged, is a measure of the complexity of modern medicine. Once the limited attempt to cure or alleviate the sickness of an individual, the art and science of medicine now forms only part of a vast endeavour to maintain all people of all ages and of all nations at the highest possible level of health.

Bibliography and further reading

General Histories of Medicine
H. Fielding Garrison, *An Introduction to the History of Medicine*. W. B. Saunders Co., Philadelphia, 4th edn, 1929.
The standard text book of medical history. Detailed, contains biographies. Little knowledge of medical terminology needed. For reference rather than for reading.

Charles Singer and E. Ashworth Underwood, *A Short History of Medicine*. Clarendon Press, Oxford, 1962.
The second edition of 1962 is a much better book than the first. An excellent account treated by subjects. Rather lengthy and considerable knowledge of medical terminology is necessary.

Douglas Guthrie, *A History of Medicine*. Thomas Nelson and Sons, London, 1945 and later editions.
A simple, interesting and reasonably full account of the history of medicine, from the earliest times, contained in just over 400 pages. Little knowledge of medical terminology required. This is probably the best introduction to the subject for the lay reader.

Chapter 1
S. G. Blaxland Stubbs and E. W. Bligh, *Sixty Centuries of Health and Physick*. Sampson Low Marston and Co., London, 1931.
Subtitled 'the progress of ideas from primitive magic to modern medicine' this lavishly illustrated work is one of the best for the general reader. Still obtainable from specialized libraries.

J. Chadwick and W. N. Mann, *The Medical Works of Hippocrates*. Blackwell, Oxford, 1950.
It is difficult to choose a suitable book from the immense amount of Hippocrates literature. This is one of the better for the general reader.

G. Sarton, *Galen of Pergamon*. University of Kansas Press, 1954.
An adequate account of Galen's life, writings and influence.

Sir T. Clifford Allbutt, *Greek Medicine in Rome*. Macmillan and Co., London, 1921.
A short book, published over fifty years ago, which is still the best account of how Greek medicine reached Rome and so influenced the remainder of Western Europe. Non-technical and can be read like a novel. Obtainable from specialist libraries.

Stanley Rubin, *Mediaeval English Medicine*. David and Charles, Newton Abbot, 1974.
In spite of the title, deals chiefly with Anglo-Saxon medicine, but is a short and simple introduction for the general reader.

K. D. Keele, *Leonardo da Vinci on Movement of the Heart and Blood*. Harvey and Blythe Ltd, London, 1952.
The subject is not so limited as suggested by the title. An excellent account of the change in medical thinking effected by the Renaissance. Some knowledge of medical terminology required, but recommended.

William Osler, *The Evolution of Modern Medicine*. Yale University Press, New Haven, 1921.
A short series of lectures by one of the greatest of medical historians and writers. Repays reading for this reason as well as for the content. Obtainable from specialized libraries.

Chapter 2
R. M. Clay, *The Mediaeval Hospitals of England*. First edition, Methuen and Co., London, 1909. Second edition, Cass and Co., London, 1966.
The fact that this book was republished half a century after the first edition indicates its worth. The only really detailed account of the subject, interesting and suitable for the lay reader. Contains a list of hospitals under place names and so is invaluable as a source for projects connected with local history.

F. N. L. Poynter (edit.), *The Evolution of Hospitals in Britain*. Pitman Medical Publishing Co., London, 1964.
Contains a number of short papers by different authors read at the biennial conference of the British Society for the History of Medicine. Provides a good over-all picture of hospital development and is recommended to the non-medical reader.

Chapter 3
C. H. Talbot and E. A. Hammond, *The Medical Practitioners in Mediaeval England*. Wellcome Medical Historical Library, London, 1965.
A series of short biographies of all traceable medical practitioners, including the few known in the Anglo-Saxon period, and ending in 1518. The story is then taken up in part by W. Munk, *The Roll of the Royal College of Physicians of London*. The index contains place names. Not for general reading but invaluable as a source book for local historical projects.

K. Pollak and E. Ashworth Underwood, *The Healers*. Thomas Nelson and Sons, Ltd, London, 1968.
A survey not only of medical ideas but of the doctors who practised them from the earliest times until the present day. Recommended for general reading.

F. N. L. Poynter (edit.), *The Evolution of Medical Practice in Britain*. Pitman Medical Publishing Co., London, 1961.
F. N. L. Poynter (edit.), *The Evolution of Medical Education in Britain*. Pitman Medical Publishing Co., London, 1966.
Both books consist of papers by various authors read at the biennial conferences of the British Society for the History of Medicine. Both

provide excellent surveys of their subjects, are not too technical, and are recommended for general reading.

Charles E. Newman, *The Evolution of Medical Education in the Nineteenth Century*. Oxford University Press, London, 1957.
A good account of the more modern period. Recommended.

Chapter 4

Charles Creighton, *A History of Epidemics in Britain*. Two volumes. Cambridge University Press, 1891.
This old book is still the standard history of epidemics. Volume I ends with the extinction of bubonic plague in Britain. A compendium of information from which much recent literature on plague derives. Suitable for the non-medical reader and obtainable from specialist libraries.

J. F. D. Shrewsbury, *A History of Bubonic Plague in the British Isles*. Cambridge University Press, 1970.
This exasperating book contains invaluable information on both national and local outbreaks of plague. Place names are given in the index. The best reference book for local historical projects. Professor Shrewsbury appears to have written his book with the set intention of disproving 'the Black Death myth'. He has been led into a number of patent absurdities and the majority of historians, medical or lay, do not accept his conclusions. Cannot be advised for general reading but contains information not easily obtainable elsewhere.

Walter George Bell, *The Great Plague in London in 1665*. John Lane at the Bodley Head, London, 1924.
Perhaps the best account. A book that well repays reading if it can be obtained.

E. P. Wilson, *The Plague in Shakespeare's London*. Oxford University Press, London, 1927. Oxford Paperbacks, 1963.
Excellent and concise account of a relatively unexplored period in the history of plague. Recommended as of special interest to the general reader.

Philip Ziegler, *The Black Death*. Collins, London, 1969 and Penguin Books, Harmondsworth, 1970.
There have been several recent studies of the Black Death, of which this is perhaps the best. Easily read and strongly recommended.

Chapter 5

Charles Creighton, *A History of Epidemics in Britain*. Two volumes. Cambridge University Press, 1891.
Contains a massive amount of information about smallpox, particularly in the second volume. Creighton seems to have been the first medical writer to understand that smallpox started to decline before the introduction of vaccination. His views on vaccination were bitterly attacked at the time of publication but now command respect.

J. D. Rolleston, *The History of the Acute Exanthemata*. William Heinemann Ltd, London, 1937.
A short but adequate historical study of smallpox, chicken pox, scarlet fever and measles written by a well-known physician. Not technical.

A. H. Gale, *Epidemic Diseases*. Penguin Books, Harmondsworth, 1959.
A concise history of all infectious diseases contained in just over 150
pages. Illustrated by graphs, largely based on the London Bills of
Mortality. Some knowledge of medical terminology is required. Gale really
contains all that the non-specialist reader needs to know about this
subject.

Dorothy Fisk, *Dr Jenner of Berkeley*. Heinemann, London, 1959.
An interesting account of Jenner's life and work which can be recommended for general reading.

Chapter 6
C. Fraser Brockington, *A Short History of Public Health*. J. and A.
Churchill Ltd, London, 1966.
A condensed but adequate history of public health from the earliest times
until 1948. Contains all the information required for ordinary purposes.
Recommended to the general reader.

C. Fraser Brockington, *Public Health in the Nineteenth Century*. E. and S.
Livingstone, Edinburgh, 1965.
An excellent and quite short description of public health work 1805–71.
Contains short biographies of John Simon's team. Recommended.

R. A. Lewis, *Edwin Chadwick and the Public Health Movement 1832–54*.
London, 1952.
An important study of Chadwick and the formative period of public
health. Recommended for general reading.

W. M. Frazer, *A History of English Public Health 1834–1939*. Baillière,
Tindall and Cox, London, 1950.
Exhaustive and largely concerned with legislation. A book for the serious
student of social history.

Donald Hunter, *Health in Industry*. Penguin Books, Harmondsworth,
1959.
A short, easy account of legislation chiefly concerning industrial disease,
poisoning and accidents. Contains all the information on this subject
required by a general reader.

H. Harold Scott, *Some Notable Epidemics*. Edward Arnold and Co.,
London, 1934.
Deals with the nineteenth and early twentieth centuries. Still one of the
best sources for the cholera epidemics. Obtainable from specialist libraries.

John Snow, *On Cholera*. Reprint of original work by Hafner, New York,
1965.
Snow's fascinating search for the cause of cholera reads like a detective
story. The book not only repays study for this reason but because it
presents a picture of mid-nineteenth century methods. Can be obtained
from a specialist library and requires no special technical knowledge.

Chapter 7
There is an immense literature on syphilis and tuberculosis. The general
reader will find sufficient for his purpose in the following:

A. H. Gale op. cit., for the history.
C. Fraser Brockington, *A Short History of Public Health* for public health measures.
W. M. Frazer op. cit., for a more detailed account of legislation and public health measures up to 1939.

Chapter 8
The rapid advance of medicine and surgery in the nineteenth century is best followed by reading one of the general histories of medicine mentioned above. The following are recommended as books of special interest on various subjects:

Charles Wilcocks, *Medical Advances, Public Health and Social Evolution*. Pergamon Press, Oxford and London, 1965.
One of the few good books on medical history written specially for school upper forms. The author is a specialist in tropical diseases and relates recent advances mainly to the problems of developing countries. He links the gradual evolution of medical thought with levels of culture and intellect in selected periods of history. Particularly relevant to the nineteenth and early twentieth centuries. Recommended for the use of teachers as well as for pupils.

W. D. Foster, *A History of Medical Bacteriology and Immunology*. William Heinemann Medical Books Ltd, London, 1970.
Good account of the development of the Germ Theory and the work in general of Louis Pasteur and Robert Koch together with more recent discoveries. Some knowledge of medical terminology needed but suitable for the lay reader.

R. J. Dubos, *Louis Pasteur Free Lance of Science*. Victor Gollancz Ltd, London, 1951.
An excellent and full account of Pasteur's work rather than of his life. Recommended for general reading.

Robert G. Richardson, *The Surgeon's Tale*. Charles Scribner's Sons, New York, 1958.
Frederick F. Cartwright, *The Development of Modern Surgery*. Arthur Barker Ltd, London, 1967.
Two rather similar books, written specially for the general reader, describing how surgery has advanced to its present state. Now out of print but obtainable from medical libraries.

Kenneth D. Keele, *The Evolution of Clinical Methods in Medicine*. Pitman Medical Publishing Co. Ltd, London, 1963.
A useful book because it describes how the doctor puts theoretical knowledge into practice. A concise account but some knowledge of medical terminology is essential.

A. R. Bleich, *The Story of X-rays from Röntgen to Isotopes*. Dover Publications Inc., New York, and Constable, London, 1960.
Deals not only with Röntgen's discovery and its application to medicine but with the use of X-rays in science and art. Contains a glossary of medical and scientific terms. A short book to be recommended.

Chapter 9

Erwin H. Ackerknecht (trans. S. Wolff), *A Short History of Psychiatry*. Hafner Publishing Co., New York and London, 1959.
A very good short history in only ninety-three pages. Suitable for the general reader.

Richard Hunter and Ida Macalpine, *Psychiatry for the Poor*. William Dawson and Sons Ltd, London, 1974.
Subtitled '1851 Colney Hatch Asylum Friern Hospital 1973' this is a fascinating history of the most famous asylum in Britain which provides a clear picture of nineteenth century conditions. A short section on types of mental disorder requires some knowledge of medical terminology. Recommended for general reading.

Brian Abel Smith, *The Hospitals 1800—1948*.
A valuable and full account of hospitals and their administration until the introduction of the National Health Service. Excellent both for reference and general reading.

G. M. Ayers, *England's First State Hospitals and the Metropolitan Asylums Board 1867—1930*. The Wellcome Historical Medical Library, London, 1971.
The development of the infirmary system. Not a book for general reading but a valuable source of information for a social history project.

Ruth G. Hodgkinson, *The Origins of the National Health Service*. The Wellcome Historical Medical Library, London, 1967.
An exhaustive account of medical services under the New Poor Law 1834—71. For the specialist reader and for reference.

Brian Watkin, *Documents on Health and Social Services 1834 to the Present Day*. Methuen and Co. Ltd, London, 1975.
The title is self-explanatory. Obviously not a book for general reading but a very convenient compendium of legislation for reference.

Chapter 10

Lindsey Almont, *Socialized Medicine in England and Wales*. The University of Carolina Press and Oxford University Press, London, 1962.
An exhaustive account of the British National Health Services 1948—61. Not a book for the general reader but of considerable interest to the social and medical historian.

Basil Druitt, *The Growth of the Welfare State*. Hamish Hamilton, London, 1966.
A short paperback, little more than a pamphlet, which contains most of the information required by a general reader, and is a useful introduction to the subject.

The First Ten Years of the World Health Organization. WHO, Geneva, 1958.
There are probably later editions of this publication but it serves as a useful reference book. Official report of WHO's work.

C. Fraser Brockington, *World Health*. Churchill Livingstone, Edinburgh, London, New York, 3rd edn, 1975 and Penguin Books, Harmondsworth.

A fine short account of problems which have been solved by WHO or which still have to be faced. This popular book is recommended as that most suitable for the general reader.

Glossary

Aetiology: Science of the causes of diseases.

Alastrim: *Variola minor*, the mild form of smallpox.

Anthrax: Disease of cattle transferable to man.

Antiseptic: Old meaning: a drug to combat developed sepsis. Modern: a drug lethal to bacteria by contact.

Antitoxin: Serum to neutralize toxic products of microorganisms.

Arteriosclerosis: 'Hardening of the arteries.'

Artificial pneumothorax: Collapse of lung by surgical means, often by injecting air or nitrogen.

Aseptic: Surgically sterile; predestruction of organisms by heat or other means.

Auscultation: Listening; medically, detection of sounds in heart and lungs by stethoscope.

Autopsy: Postmortem examination of body.

Bacillus: A rod-like bacterium.

Bacterium: Microscopic unicellullar organism.

Biochemistry: Chemistry of body constituents.

Cadaver: Corpse. Term generally used in anatomy.

Capillary network: Junction (anastomosis) of minute peripheral veins and arteries.

Cirrhosis: 'Hobnail Liver' commonly, but not always, associated with chronic alcoholic excess.

Coronary infarction: Clot in the blood vessels supplying the heart muscle. Termed 'syncope' until twentieth century.

Cowpox: Disease of cattle transmissible by contact to man.

Cretinism: Retarded mental and physical development caused by deficiency of thyroid secretion.

Crookes' Tube: Lamp producing beam of cathode rays or stream of electrons.

Delirium tremens: 'The Horrors': acute alcoholism accompanied by shaking limbs and delusions, often visual, e.g. pink rats.

Diathesis: Obsolescent term meaning a constitutional predisposition to a disease.

Disease: Endemic, occurring sporadically but continuously in a certain area or community.

Epidemic, prevalent in a community at a certain time.

Exotic, introduced from one community to another.

Pandemic, prevalent over a whole community or the world.

Droplet infection: Infection transmitted by spray from talking, coughing or sneezing.

Dysentery: Water-borne disease affecting the intestines.

Eczema: Common skin disease of several kinds.

Efflorescence: 'Bursting into flower.' Reddening of the skin seen around a healing wound or an infection such as a boil.

Elective: Term used by old surgeons to denote any operation not undertaken as an emergency or life-saving measure.

Embryology: Science of the embryo, now loosely used as the science of development.

Epidemiology: Science of epidemics, generalized into the study of infectious diseases.

Erysipelas: 'St Anthony's Fire.' An infection causing bright red colour of the skin.

Filaria: Thread-like worms which can cause tropical elephantiasis.

Galenical: A medicament compounded of several herbs or other ingredients.

Gene: Factor or element transmitted by parent to offspring.

General Paralysis: 'GPI.' An end result of syphilis often characterized by delusions of grandeur or other gross character change.

Geriatric: Pertaining to old age.

Germ: Obsolete term for any microorganism, particularly one causing disease.

Great Pox: Old term for the major skin eruption of syphilis.

Histology: Science of tissues; particularly applied to microscopical differentiation between one tissue, normal or abnormal, and another.

Humour: One of the four body fluids, water, blood, phlegm or bile.

Hypochondria, Hysteria: In ancient medical terminology have the same meaning of apparently causeless ill-health or functional disturbance, hypochondria in the male and hysteria in the female.

Iatrogenic: A horrible neologism implying disease caused by the physician; more often applied to side-effects of the drugs which he administers.

Immunity: Acquired or hereditary, partial or complete resistance to an infection.

Infantile diarrhoea: Summer diarrhoea, infantile cholera: one of the chief causes of high infant mortality especially in the summer months. Last major outbreak in 1911. The cause is not certainly known.

Inguinal: Of the groin.

Inoculation: Injection of organisms of disease, modified by some means, to protect by a harmless or mild attack.

King's Evil: Tuberculosis of glands, particularly in the neck. Often called scrofula, but scrofula included tuberculosis of bones and joints.

Lazar: Originally any poor and diseased person. Later applied to a leper. Thence lazar-house, a place of confinement for lepers. So to lazaretto, a quarantine hospital or ship.

Leech: This very interesting term derives from the Old English *laece* meaning a healer. Thence applied to the blood-sucking insect often used by the healer. In eighteenth and nineteenth centuries came a reversal, the name of the blood-sucking insect being used as a derogatory term for any doctor. Leech or Leach is the only common English surname derived from the trade of medicine, although variations of Apothecary are very occasionally found.

Lesion: Demonstrable change caused by a disease process.

Ligation: Tying; used particularly by surgeons for securing the cut end of a blood-vessel.

Lithotomy: 'Cutting for the stone.' Removal of a bladder stone.

Lock Hospital: Hospital for treatment of venereal disease.

Lymph: Clear exudate, especially from the vesicles of cowpox.

Media: Used in medical terminology to denote nutritive broths or jellies for culture of bacteria.

Mesmerism: Hypnotism, animal magnetism; induction of a trance or actual sleep by a second person.

Miasma: A noxious emanation carried in and by the air.

Microorganism: Any living being which cannot be seen except by magnification.

Microtome: Instrument used in microscopy for cutting very thin sections.

Morphology: Science of the form of animals and plants.

Mutation: Genetic change tending towards the production of a new species.

Obstetric: Probably originated as a term to imply the science underlying the practice of midwifery. The two words now have virtually the same meaning.

Orthopaedic: Literally, correction of childhood deformities. Now applied to the surgery of bones and joints.

Ovariotomy: Puncture or actual removal of a cyst of the ovary. The only common abdominal operation performed by the pre-Listerian surgeon.

Paediatric: Pertaining to children; in medical terminology refers more to the special care and treatment of children than to childhood diseases.

Patella: Knee-cap.

Pathogenic: Causing disease; particularly of bacteria. That is, pathogenic bacteria cause disease, non-pathogenic are harmless or beneficial.

Pathology: Implies the science of disease. Now used in the more restricted sense of laboratory rather than bedside diagnosis.

Percussion: Method of tapping with the finger to ascertain areas of relative dullness and resonance, particularly in the chest.

Petri dish: Glass plate (? now plastic) covered with nutrient medium for culture of bacteria.

Phagocyte: 'Eating cell.' Large white blood corpuscle which ingests foreign bodies such as bacteria.

Pharmacopoeia: List of drugs with directions for use. 'Materia Medica' is properly the drugs listed in a pharmacopoeia.

Phthisis: Old term for pulmonary tuberculosis or consumption.

Physiology: Science of normal function.

Plastic surgery: Repair of structural deficiencies; *not* simple skin-grafting.

Pock mark: The scar left by a smallpox pustule.

Prophylactic: Any measure tending to prevent disease.

Psychotic: Antithesis of somatic; psychotic disease is an illness or disorder of the mind not due to an apparent organic cause. Now more usually 'psychiatric' which properly implies the treatment given or the attendant physician.

Puerperal fever: Generalized infection during the puerperum, i.e. infection following childbirth.

Pus: Product of infection, particularly an infected wound. 'Laudable pus' is that produced by a local infection. Locally infected wounds were so common that 'laudable pus' was thought to be an essential stage of healing until the nineteenth century.

Pythogenic theory: Later term for the theory of miasma. The derivation is obscure, but probably refers to the great snake of Delphi killed by Apollo. In mythology disease is often represented by a snake.

Regimen: Old term for prescribed course of treatment, including diet and exercises.

Resistance: Natural body defence against disease, particularly against invasion by pathogenic organisms.

Resuscitation: Restoration to a state compatible with continued life. Now often 'intensive care'.

Saprophyte: Organism living on dead or decayed matter, animal or vegetable.

Scab: Natural protective crust of dried blood and exudate which forms a barrier to bacteria and under which wound healing can take place.

Serum: The liquid part of the blood from which the corpuscles have been removed. Often used loosely to imply serum containing antitoxins for therapeutic use.

Shock: A clinical entity (pallor, sweating, lowered blood pressure) usually associated with blood loss but also with other causes such as acute pain.

Simple: A single herb. Cf. *Galenical*, a compound mixture.

Somatic: Pertaining to the body. Physical or organic disease.

Suppuration: Production of pus; festering.

Tabes: Locomotor ataxia; one of the terminal phases of syphilis.

Temperaments: The four types of constitution derived from excess of one of the four humours: melancholic (water), sanguine (blood), phlegmatic (phlegm), choleric (bile).

Therapeutics: Science of treatment of disease.

Trepanning: Or trephining; cutting a circular piece from the skull.

Typhoid: A water-borne fever very prevalent in the nineteenth century.

Typhus: Spotted fever; probably the famine-sickness of ancient records. Tends to occur in such conditions. For example, in the Irish Potato Famines and in Russia during the Civil War.

Vaccine: The term commemorates Jenner's vaccination, but is now applied to preventive inoculation with dead or modified organisms of various types.

Vaccinia: Properly *Variola vaccinae*, cowpox. More commonly used as 'generalized vaccinia', a rare and dangerous illness following vaccination.

Variolation: Inoculation with matter derived from a smallpox pustule.

Virus: A minute microorganism, smaller than a bacterium, capable of causing a disease of which smallpox is one example.

Wise woman: Probably originally a white witch, became applied to a midwife and to a person particularly skilled in the sick-care of babies.

Index

Index